GW00703038

Just a Bang on the Head

To my Gran, Pearl Emily Neal, who taught me the value of courage, determination and having a passion for life and to my mother, Eileen, who never stood in my way and always kept loving me.

Just a Bang on the Head

Living with a Brain Injury

Rosie Belton

craig potton publishing

First published in 2008 by Craig Potton Publishing

Craig Potton Publishing
98 Vickerman Street, PO Box 555, Nelson, New Zealand
www.craigpotton.co.nz

Text © Rosie Belton

ISBN 978-1-877333-77-4

Printed in Wellington by Astra Print Ltd

This book is copyright. Apart from any fair dealing for the purposes of private study, research, criticism or review, as permitted under the Copyright Act, no part may be reproduced by any process without the permission of the publishers.

Author's Note

Since my brain injury, in February 2004, I have written as often as I could. It has been very challenging and emotionally gruelling to have to relive the journey each time I edited or changed things around. One day during the second year I decided I would call where I was at with my writing an ending, and send it off to a publisher. This was a frightening task, especially because the whole procedure was new for me. After a working lifetime spent in one medium – the drama and theatre world – here I was stepping out into completely unknown territory, opening myself to criticism and rejection. But what did I have to lose? Nothing compared with the possible gains: first, of achieving completion of a project; and, second, of getting out there what I kept continuing to experience, writing words that might provide comfort for, or find resonance with, others in a similar situation.

Although the manuscript wasn't accepted immediately, some of the feedback from a potential publisher and some very practical suggestions to get editing assistance encouraged me. I needed a break from the closeness of this project, so I welcomed neutral and professional input. My writing had started to become a book. It scared me that this was my journey, in print – this was me and my family and my friends, my therapists and my assistants. I felt exposed and nervous about sharing this with strangers, and I found it even more disturbing that this journey I was on wasn't yet over.

Foreword

Just a Bang on the Head is a vigorous and revealing text about the damaging and often cruel effects of brain injury. Thousands of people in New Zealand, Australia and nearby Asia experience brain injury and are hidden from our view, and certainly from our understanding. The community does not know about them. Their condition is often not immediately observed, let alone realised. They are forgotten people.

Rosie Belton's story doesn't spare the reader, and it shouldn't if we are to realise the nature and extent of this hidden disability. Rosie makes clear the sense of loss experienced by people with brain injury: their memory loss, their disorientation, their loss of physical strength and difficulty controlling emotions and, ultimately, their humiliation. Vulnerability following brain injury permeates the pages. And all this resulted suddenly from a fall and a bang on the head while dancing. *Just a Bang on the Head* is a substantive and insightful autobiographical text that has a necessary message for us all. You don't return to your former self when you experience brain injury.

Three years after her accident, Rosie tells of persisting punishing noise sensitivity, vertigo problems and visual disturbance. These effects don't just disappear. But throughout all this Rosie remains resilient and positive, equipped with a determination to keep pushing herself. *Just a Bang on the Head* is about trialling every possible means of recovery — a formidable task and achievement.

This is a story of loss, courage and adjustment. It is also a social medicine story about the fine detail necessary for effective rehabilitation. Rosie's story needs to be read by the general public as well as by medical practitioners, teachers and allied health professionals who work with people who have experienced brain injury and comparable neurological disorders. This is because *Just a Bang on the Head* not only reveals the long-term neurological and social effects of brain injury but also the never-ending rehabilitation and adjustment, in which the benefits of human touch underpin Rosie's struggle to hang on to parts of her former life, while keeping intellectually active, yet not over-stimulated.

Reading this story provides one with a glimpse of the debilitating effects of the hidden disability of brain injury. It is a story that could easily happen to any one of us tomorrow, yet the recovery process, demonstrated so succinctly and openly by Rosie, is a lifelong process, tapping personal resilience and creativity.

Roger J Rees
Rehabilitation Consultant
Emeritus Professor: Disability Research
School of Medicine, Flinders University
Adelaide, Australia

Prologue

I t's spring. It's my birthday and the house is rich with the scent of flowers. I'm trying to describe to my husband, Mark, how I'm feeling: grateful to be alive, yes, but frustrated that the recovery is so slow.

For years during my busy 'other' life – the one before this – I used to say to myself and sometimes to others that one day, when I had time, I would begin to collate the writing I'd done over the years. Well, I have time now – plenty of it. But what I'm writing about isn't exactly what I'd planned.

This was the old life, according to the CV: director/producer for twenty-five years in theatre production, film and television; casting agent and director; drama tutor (youth and adult students); lecturer; teacher of drama studies; founder/director of a drama school; tutor workshop facilitator; drama trainer for medical students (interpersonal and self-development); New Zealand delegate for an international young people's theatre organisation; and a working Director in my husband's business.

I was a mother of three, a grandmother of four, a wife, the manager of a busy household and large garden in Governors Bay on Banks Peninsula, about twenty minutes from Christchurch city. Mobility – local, national and international – was an accepted fact of life.

But then a bang on the head changed everything.

One

The weather had been particularly unsettled and cool – a bit worrying for my friend's daughter, who was getting married outside. But 7 February 2004 dawned grey and clear. I was awake early, knowing I must sew the fresh rosebuds onto the mosquito netting designed to hang from a tree over the four-tiered wedding cake.

For me it was the end of an extremely busy two months. Children and grandchildren had been with us for an extended period. From Patagonia, Queensland and New Zealand they had arrived, filling the house and garden with the joy and chaos different generations bring. Despite the odd problem, it had been a precious time of richness and connection, especially watching the little ones – part of us – in our environment.

I loved these early hours of the morning before the smallest person in the household woke. It took a long time and lots of patience, of which I have little, to get the tiny Cecile Brunner buds and the deep blue hydrangea petals sewn onto the net. Once this task was completed, I laid out my silk outfit and contemplated which shoes to wear – the high ones, sent recently by a friend in Sydney, which matched perfectly but looked, and felt, as if they could be most uncomfortable when worn for many hours; or the lower, more practical ones? I chose the high ones for the church service and decided I would change into the others for the reception. That seemed a practical solution.

The day went by as planned: a visit to the hairdresser – the bob cut full and bouncy – then to the day spa for a pedicure, manicure and my make-up. Finally, I went off to pick up the pearls that would add the finishing touch to my outfit. It was raining a little as I left town, but not enough to ruin the celebrations. The rest of the family had their various jobs – on cameras and gates. Mark and I set out for what promised to be a great day.

Two

It was around 11 PM. The dancing was full on. The band members, musos from our past, offered rhythms and beats that all the age groups present could respond to. I was rock and rolling with a vibrant, youthful partner. I remember thinking, My heart is really pumping fast: I haven't danced this fast and this long for quite a while – I hope I don't collapse! Since seeing *They Shoot Horses, Don't They?* years before, I'd always thought that if I had to 'go' in an accident, dancing for me would be an acceptable 'what' and a gorgeous outdoor venue would be quite an acceptable 'where'. I've always loved to dance, for the freedom it gives and the joy it brings, and for the unspoken connection with your partner, the concentration on finding a pattern between you. The silk skirt moved beautifully.

What I remember next is my heels coming into contact with the flower bucket placed to protect dancers from the outdoor tap, feeling myself airborne momentarily, shocked to be so, and then the back of my head making contact with the earth as I fell. My partner was soon beside me, pulling me to my feet. I felt that my brain had been jolted inside my skull. I thought I heard a sound inside my head. I cried with the shock of it, and the pain – because there was instantaneous pain. People seemed to find the incident amusing – it was late, it was party time, and we were clowning around.

Nothing a bit of Chardonnay and a few more wild dances wouldn't fix. And that's what I did. I went into a renewed frenzy of dancing and even a spot of stage singing with a few other participants. But the pain remained. Nothing made it go away.

The next day, I woke with the sickening pain that stayed with me for the next five weeks. Panadol during the day, a Chardonnay in the evenings and plenty of determined distraction kept me from dwelling on my situation.

But stranger and stranger things began to happen to me.

Three

It had been a full-on summer. My energy levels had been pushed to their limits over and over again. My stress levels, too, were incredibly high – I had business and money worries, a constant nagging feeling that I wasn't achieving my own goals separate from the family, and then just the ordinary fatigue from running a large household for a lot of people.

When the symptoms began to harass me, I thought, Oh well, these are messages telling me to slow down. The first thing I did, around 9 February, was to ring the osteopath. Perhaps the fall had put my back out. I couldn't get an appointment for three days, so I said I'd call back if I needed to. Maybe a massage would be a good thing, but I didn't get around to booking it. The week was incredibly busy. My daughter, Aimee, and her family had left the week before the wedding, and my son Mischa, his partner Sol and their almost-one-year-old, my darling youngest grandchild, Lili, were leaving in two weeks' time.

We had so much to do – get Lili's birthday party ready, and help them to buy a car, pack and ready themselves for a shift to another part of the country. They had decided to stay on in New Zealand for longer and perhaps do some seasonal work here before returning to Argentina, so there were air tickets to change and immigration paperwork to deal with. In between all this, I had to go to the offices – both Mark's and mine. The week before the party on the 14th went by in a bit of a blur. There was a lot of pain but I kept going. The party was wonderful: about ten children and fifteen adults, delicious food, a thunderstorm in the middle and a piñata to break open on the patio.

I kept going. Things got stranger. My left hand had become weakened in a very subtle way. I would, for example, be driving the car and go to park it. I would pull on the handbrake, get out of the car and then glance back to see it moving. I hadn't secured the brake. Confused, I would open the door and lean back into the car to pull the brake on again. This happened more than once. It left me increasingly puzzled. One day, when holding a glass of wine, I saw the glass tilt and begin to spill. Why was that happening? I didn't seem to have anything to do with the action. The same thing happened with a plate of food. If I held it with my left hand it would tilt very gently, more and more. I mentioned these occurrences, of course, to Mark, and laughed about them. How odd.

We entertain fairly regularly and I found myself doing very uncharacteristic things. For example, I'm usually very organised, planning at least a day ahead, purchasing appropriate groceries and so on. My cousin and family, who live nearby, had an overseas visitor and we'd arranged for us all to have a meal at our place before the last of our family visitors departed.

The week had been filled with packing and sorting, so, for a treat, on the afternoon before the meal my daughter-in-law and I went to the spa – a leg wax for her, a facial for me. I thought it would relax me, make me feel better, take the pain away. But no, it was awful – I felt terrible during the facial, and worse later. My face felt weird down one side, kind of numb, and my ear hurt at times. The head pains were fairly constant. Ordinary things seemed very difficult. I was tired, and I couldn't seem to get everything done. I felt a bit vacant. Knowing that something wasn't right, I didn't commit to making the whole meal for the ten or twelve of us. My responsibility was to get the table set, and to make the focaccia bread, the dips and the dessert. My cousin's family would bring pizza, and Mischa, who is a wonderful pizza maker, said he would supply another.

Both our spa appointments were running late. When I looked at my watch and saw the time I knew rationally there was no way I could get home and cook, set a table and get the house ready for guests. And for the first time in my life I didn't care. There seemed to be no link between the reality of time and the reality of the invitation I had extended; I experienced no guilt, made no attempt to sort it out – I simply accepted that the situation was impossible to solve.

And so we drove home. It was chaos. The guests had arrived and were probably shocked by my change of behaviour. I think I managed to set a table. My son made a couple of pizzas at high speed, and the visitors readied the kitchen and dining table for ten hungry people. I felt odd during the evening but put it down to the facial having stirred something up.

Four

Jetlag without the travel – that's how it felt. My closest female friend, Sarah, was away for a few weeks so I hadn't been able to talk to her. I was beginning to feel more and more of a failure. I wasn't coping, and my husband was facing increasing business challenges. Then Michelle, our wonderful temp at work, announced she had to leave and move on, as she wanted to see some more of New Zealand before her work visa ran out. We advertised for a new part-time office administrator and I turned myself to the task of sorting and sifting through the applications. I short-listed about five or six and Michelle rang them to set up interview times. My usual confidence in carrying out such a task was diminishing, but so very subtly that I couldn't be definitive about it.

My coping mechanisms were changing – I became sleepy, less acute. I was fluctuating in my behaviour and probably acting quite inappropriately. My husband seemed too busy to help, so I floated on. During the interviews I felt as though I was encased in cotton wool. My usual decisiveness was leaving me. I would promise one person something, then promise the next one the same. I would say I'd call, then fail to do so. I would be animated, then flat. What must those interviewees have thought of me?

There was one girl, the youngest of those we recalled, who had potential. She possessed abilities that, with guidance and supervision, meant she would grow into the job, and because she was so young she would adapt to a new situation if the business didn't pull out of its nosedive and we had to let her go. We offered her the position. In retrospect, this was the most ridiculous decision: she couldn't support me in our critical situation – she was the one who needed support and guidance.

By now the days were becoming blurred. My son and his family were packing and about to go north. There were houses to find, and jobs. There was the new girl at work to mentor, the house and property to run, and auditions coming up for the extras I was to find to appear in the film of *The Lion, the Witch and the Wardrobe*. I wasn't coping and my husband seemed unable to hear or see.

The nights were so long. I couldn't lie flat because my head felt it had so much pressure in it.

Packed into their newly purchased old white Toyota Corona, my son and his family drove off to fresh adventures in Nelson. As they drove up Sandy Beach Road, the car almost scraping the ground at the gate with its extra weight, I prayed that they would have a safe journey and successful months ahead in their new home.

When I turned back towards the house, I felt I was going to die from exhaustion. The pain was unbelievably bad. Somehow I stumbled into the house, face awash with tears, and put myself to bed. That was about 10 AM on Saturday, the 27th of February. For the next three days I hardly got out of bed except to drag together some meals and have hot baths. I think at some stage Mark took me to the pictures.

He was distracted and preoccupied, locking himself away in his office at home. I thought I was crashing because the long summer of work for the family had suddenly come to a close, but when I finally got going again, probably on about March the 1st, I felt no better. Now I knew I must see a doctor. I made an appointment for the 4th. I felt so confused, equating my state with failure as a mother, as a wife, as a business partner. The business situation was getting increasingly bad. The new girl was to start on the 10th or

11th, and there would be just two days of crossover before Michelle left. I remember waking up in the mornings after extremely broken sleep and thinking I might as well finish things. I was no good to anyone, I felt so bad. I contemplated just walking into the sea and not stopping. I longed to feel the water close over me and to drift away from the pain and the weird feelings, to get away from the conflict in my life, from the fears and worries.

It was the last two weeks in New Zealand for Emily, my youngest son Ollie's girlfriend at the time; she was relocating overseas. I wanted to have her to dinner. Ollie rang to say they could come on Wednesday the 10th, which was the only free evening they both had.

On top of all this I'd been invited to attend a meeting in Warsaw to discuss drama methods and their usefulness in education, and to speak about my experiences as an educator using drama methods. This was the part of my work in which I was most passionately interested, so I had accepted. The flights had been booked and accommodation arrangements in Poland completed. I was to give a presentation about my work over the past twenty years, using drama as a tool for learning in New Zealand. It was an exciting opportunity to tie all that experience together. I'd never visited Poland before, though I knew the Polish organisers from previous conferences.

But something was wrong – and more than the fact that money was a problem. I just didn't feel confident enough to actually purchase the tickets. I lacked my usual drive to make an itinerary and secure a hotel room en route in Singapore. I was uncharacteristically anxious. My travel agent indulged me: she stretched out the payment date. I promised the organisers in Poland that I was onto it, that yes, I would give the presentation, and that yes, I would take the accommodation offered.

I was supposed to fly out on March the 12th. On the 4th I finally saw my doctor. She was compassionate about my symptoms but puzzled. I suppose I presented quite well – I can't remember. Nothing was resolved and no further action was taken. She urged me to go to Poland. 'It will distract you and inspire you,' she said, 'take you away from all the work problems your husband's experiencing.' Okay, I thought, okay. But something still stopped me from making the payment, and from doing any preparation on the paper I was to give.

On Friday the 6th I was to go to Nelson with Mark. I remember sitting waiting for him outside his office, with our large dog Bella, a Labrador/Newfoundland cross. I'd tidied the house, packed the bags, sorted all the animals and now there I was, at 6 PM, waiting. I was dreading the car trip: I had such enormous headaches, nausea, sensitivity to sound. It was hell. No one listened, especially not my busy husband. I knew I must have a back-up plan for a place to stay on the way, so I rang a B&B place I knew in Blenheim. 'Gino, have you got a room tonight for my husband and me? We'll be late, very late.' The wonderful Gino was very soothing. 'Of course, of course, don't worry. I will have a room ready and the door will be open…' So at least that was sorted.

At 6.15 PM we finally left Christchurch, me cowering with pain and distress. We dropped Bella off at the kennels; I had a row with Mark; then we were on the road north. Bumps were a nightmare, as were bright lights. I craved salt and water, so we stopped in Cheviot for salty chips and tea. I was so ill I couldn't even get out of the car. Then on to Kaikoura. I knew I had to eat, but it was so late.

Packing had been a nightmare. Here I was, a woman who had travelled and packed efficiently for years, yet I couldn't seem to coordinate such a simple task. The result had been mismatched clothing that was inappropriate for the weather, but Mark didn't seem to notice.

The stop in Kaikoura was odd. I'd always been the one who could quickly find an eating place, decide and go for it. But that night I felt unsure of myself. Mark waited in the car while I went in and returned to report that it was noisy and busy but maybe okay. I went back in, found a table and Mark finally followed after a phone call or two. I wasn't coping with the noise. Then we were informed that there was at least a twenty-minute wait. No, I couldn't stand that and nor could Mark. After two or three more places where the noise was intolerable and we would have to wait, we finally found a quiet place where they could serve us. The Panadol was kicking in – a meal and a Chardonnay and we were back on the road, with Mark driving and me dozing intermittently.

At midnight we reached Blenheim and Gino's, and the deliciousness of smooth linen and a hot bubbly bath. I was absolutely crazy with exhaustion but, as was becoming the pattern of late, could not sleep. I complained frequently to Mark, who regularly told me I was becoming emotionally manipulative, equating my increasing complaints with a reaction to his excessive workload.

Wild passion, then another sleepless night. Breakfast, as usual at Gino's, was magnificent, and with my morning Panadol taken, I could cope. But something was wrong, and I was beginning to acknowledge this. What was I to do about it? I didn't know.

Five

In Nelson, people noticed that I looked different. 'You look sad,' said my daughter-in-law Sol. 'Your face is sad.' I thought I looked different, but sad, no. What would I be sad about? My smile was odd. Always a bit crooked, it now seemed extremely so. I began to have problems putting lipstick on. My God, what was happening to me? I was starting to struggle with my clothes. Putting a bra on and doing up the hooks was becoming a nightmare. Everything was so slow and so difficult.

My mother-in-law, a retired medical practitioner, was to have afternoon tea with me at my son's home, and I was considering speaking to her as I was by now quite sure there was something seriously wrong with me. My moods were strange. I couldn't enjoy my darling Lili, who wasn't able to understand why her 'Ganga' seemed so uninterested. I just wanted to rest and rest.

That morning – it must have been March the 7th – I was having a shower and wondering about my left hand and how peculiar it felt. I was favouring my right hand more and more. I started to do a drama exercise that requires brain–hand coordination and dexterity. The neurological people would later jokingly call it 'the Rosie indicator'. It requires holding a hand up, fingers together but outstretched, then separating the fingers one at a time – little finger first, and so on. The process is then reversed. After years of doing this little exercise with students, I was very adept at it with both hands – usually.

But that day in the shower at Mischa and Sol's it didn't happen with my left hand. No message got through. I remember standing there – it was the moment of acceptance that something was terribly wrong.

A feeling of sadness and loss began to seep through me. I dried myself and got dressed. Dressing was becoming so difficult that I'd taken to wearing a 'uniform'. I wasn't conscious of choosing this outfit, but in retrospect I realise it was the most practical in the circumstances.

First, I pulled on stretch white trousers recently rescued from Gino's B&B in Blenheim, where they had been since November. Gino had rung in February to say that he was in Christchurch with some white trousers he believed I'd left behind. I denied all knowledge of these trousers, insisting they weren't mine. It was only when we got to Blenheim and he showed them to me that I realised they did indeed belong to me and that they were a very special pair at that – purchased in June in Queensland. How could I have forgotten them? It was a mystery to me. Anyway, they served the purpose now – perfect for my current deteriorating situation. On my top half I wore a loose-fitting tunic dress, with no zips and no buttons. I was adapting to my new situation, using my right side as much as I could.

The eye problem was another mystery. This had begun probably three or four weeks earlier. It was my right eye that was affected. When I was tired it would close without any will on my part. Not only that, but when I woke up in the night it would stay shut. It wasn't an infection: the eye was dry but simply refused to open. After splashing on water and making a few attempts at opening it, I would finally succeed. One night I sat up very late in order to edit the tapes of the wedding and the summer with the family. Mark had gone to bed. It must have been around 11.30 PM. I was sitting on a stool close to the TV monitor and the tape editing was going smoothly. The next thing I knew I was waking up on the floor with my eye jammed shut. I was disoriented, the screen was blank and screaming static at me. My watch said it was 1.30 AM. I struggled to my feet, turned things off and made my way to bed, confused.

It was even stranger the next day when I went to label the tapes and thought I would just quickly flick through them to check the quality. It was then that I discovered that the one I'd been working on the night before was blank — wiped. It must have happened when I'd passed out: it had taped to the end, rewound itself, then re-recorded, wiping the tape.

On March the 8th Mark cancelled my Polish trip at my request and the next day my mother-in-law asked how I was — she said I looked tired. I told her I was suffering from bad headaches and that I'd had a fall. She asked me to walk for her in a straight line. She then asked me to hold a piece of paper between my fingers and hold on when she pulled: my right hand behaved; the left didn't. She seemed concerned and told me I should see a doctor back in Christchurch. She also spoke to Mark, alerting him to her worries.

We stayed in Nelson until late in the afternoon so that we could have an early celebration for our grandson Reuben's eighth birthday. I felt awful, and on the drive back to Christchurch on Tuesday the 9th I became worse and worse. By the time we stopped in Hanmer for the night I was very pale and sick with pain. The Chardonnay and Panadol trick wasn't always working now. I was very upset and Mark was tired of me being upset.

My new work at the Christchurch Medical School didn't start for another two weeks or so. My pilot programme — teaching communication techniques to fifth-year medical students using drama methods to enhance their practice skills — had been accepted and I should have been happy, but I felt that I was merely existing. I hardly slept that night in Hanmer and woke early. It was Wednesday, 10 March. Mark wanted to work for a few hours before we left, so

I thought I would have a swim. The hot pools would do me good, I rationalised, perhaps combined with a few vigorous lengths in the cold pool. I was still terribly pale and felt extremely nauseous.

As I walked across the road to the pool entrance I felt as though I were encased in fluff – nothing was quite real. In the changing room I really struggled with my clothes. The bikini had me in despair: I just couldn't get the straps attached. I'd never felt old – was this what it was like? I was so out of control and useless.

Finally, I made it out to the pool area. Hot pool first, I thought, so in I went, but it felt very uncomfortable, not at all safe or right. I'm going crazy, I thought. This stress with Mark's work has affected me. I need to be distracted – I'll try the cold pool. I'd brought my basket of clothing and valuables with me to the pool side. This wasn't something I would normally do, but coping with a locker was just too hard. Putting my basket on the seat at the edge of the water, I went in. The cold water was a shock, but then I began – or tried to begin – swimming.

The strangest thing occurred: my right arm began to do breast-stroke, my preferred swimming method, but my left arm was like a dwarf limb. It made only the tiniest movements, causing me to be completely unbalanced and humiliated. I was distressed that people might be watching me. Very upset, I climbed out of the pool and couldn't see my basket. Fear and paranoia took over. Someone's stolen it, I thought. Then, observing my distress, one of the pool attendants showed me where the basket was – blown a few metres away by the strong, gusty nor'wester.

Picking up my basket, I returned uncertainly to the changing room. There, standing shivering on the cold concrete, I tried to manage the job of getting my bikini off and my clothes on. I never enjoy the public display of bodies in swimming pool changing rooms – I usually like to be as discreet and rapid as possible. But this day I simply couldn't get it together. Eventually, I took the bikini off, but then I couldn't get my briefs on. When I finally achieved this,

I couldn't manage my bra. I felt hopeless and humiliated. Tugging on the tunic top, I made my way miserably back to the hotel. The wind was hot and strong; I was crying and struggling – everything just seemed to require the most enormous effort.

Back at the hotel I saw myself in the mirror, ashen and pale. What was the matter with me? Mark rang my doctor, who said she would see me at 1.40 PM in Christchurch. Mark was distracted – he still had things to do before we left – so after sorting out my clothing, I went to the dining room to drink tea and try to read the paper. Then Mark came in and asked me if I would drive as he had papers to read. 'It will do you good,' he added, 'to be distracted.' I could hear what he was thinking: You're so emotional at the moment. I didn't want to drive but maybe it would be good for me.

Six

It was weird. I lacked confidence to go over eighty kilometres per hour. I lost my temper when I felt a driver was overtaking dangerously. I felt detached – on the outside looking in. Mark read and read and read. I tried to concentrate. I was frightened of cars too close to me. I'd always been poor at judging distances but today it was much worse than usual. Occasionally Mark would raise his head and say, 'Put your foot down', or 'Come on, overtake now. What's the matter with you?' It was a very uncomfortable experience. I was only just hanging on, though to what or why I didn't know.

And then at last we were coming into Christchurch. I was exhausted but Mark had no time to come with me to the doctor – he had an appointment at work, so I had to drop him at his office. There was no time, either, to pick up Bella from the kennels. I'd have to do that later. So I drove to the doctor's, arriving about 1.30 PM. When I attempted to park the car my first try was crooked. On my second try the brake wasn't on properly and I drifted out to the centre of the turnaround area. I had a third go – damn it, that would have to do. There didn't seem to be any way to make the parking better, so in I went.

'I'm no better than last week,' I told her, 'worse in fact.' I explained about the headaches, about my hand, my smile, the swimming and my mother-in-law's concerns. She tested me again for reflexes, pupil dilation, gripping abilities, walking in a straight line, heel and toe.

I could sense her concern. She referred me to the neurological unit at the hospital for a scan as soon as possible. If I hadn't heard anything by the next day, Thursday, 11 March, I was to ring her, and if other symptoms appeared at any time I was to get hold of her. I left the surgery relieved that something was being done, but distressed at how bad I felt.

Surely my friend Sarah must be back by now from the Chathams. I'd call in to see. I can't think why I didn't call my daughter in Australia. I drove to Governors Bay in a haze, very upset, and went straight to Sarah's, hoping so much that she would be there. She wasn't. Very depressed, I drove home, had a shower and took ages to get dressed. I tried to unpack and was unable to, so put on my favourite dress and applied my make-up. This took me an hour: I seemed to be swimming in a mist. I drove back to town, to Mark's office, where I tried to sort out some work problems, but I just couldn't do it.

Ollie rang to confirm that he and Emily were coming for a meal. It was now 5 PM so it would have to be a Thai takeaway. I ordered the food, then floated/rolled/dreamed my way down in the lift. Mark and I collected the food, then drove home, where our friend Philip, Sarah's husband, was waiting in the driveway. Great, now we would find out how long it would be before she returned.

It was good to see Philip. A bottle of wine was opened – a lovely Pinot – glasses were poured and the catch-up began. I attempted to set the table but couldn't manage the cloth. 'Philip,' I asked, 'is my mouth crooked? Does my face look different?' He laughed and assured me I looked the same to him. People helped me as I struggled with the impossible task of opening the plastic pottles of Thai food.

Seven

11 MARCH, 4 AM. *Disintegration almost complete. I have felt increasingly nauseous and debilitated. My work has become increasingly shambolic. Very strange to be me and still look like me, and think like me but have a body that does not behave as me.*

I muddled my way through Thursday, March the 11th. Mark left first thing for Auckland. I managed some administration work for Mark's business in the morning, then some for my office in the afternoon. A meeting with a colleague from the medical school was scheduled for later in the day. Then Philip and I planned to do something – a film, maybe, or dinner. The day was difficult. No one had rung from the hospital about the scan.

Bella was still at the kennels and I knew I must pick her up. But it all seemed so difficult. I was *so* tired. On at least two occasions I actually caught myself napping at the traffic lights.

Somewhere around 4 PM I stopped struggling to make sense of the paper war in the office and headed off to collect Bella. She was a fit young dog, weighing forty-five kilograms, and in my exhausted state I was frightened by her enthusiasm and quite unable to cope. I got her into the back seat and tied her to the seat belt. I remember having a bizarre conversation with a girl at the kennels about Bella going on heat. Then I rang Philip – I needed to touch base with someone. Where was Ollie? Probably at university. I told Philip I didn't want to stay in town – I would go home and perhaps go out with him later. I just had to get home. With Bella panting and puffing eagerly behind me, I set off on the drive to Governors Bay. Everything began to seem like a dream. The roads, so familiar, became jumbled. I wasn't sure where to go – so I just pointed the car towards the hills.

Bella strained on her leash, wanting to smother me with large doggy licks. She smelt terrible after a week in the kennels. It was just before the Blenheim Road junction that I found myself dozing off. It was like jetlag: I couldn't keep awake. I pinched myself and tried to take deep breaths. Suddenly there was a puff of air inside the car. Bewildered, I woke up to realise that Bella had stood on the window controls. By straining forward she could just place her feet on the panel between the two front seats and all four windows had shot down. The rush of breeze got me going again.

The lights changed and the traffic moved off, me with it, in a dream. I was now on the short bit of motorway leading towards Cashmere and Halswell, amid cars travelling at 100 kilometres per hour. As I made my way into the right-hand lane, I slowed down, knowing I would be taking an exit soon. I was being overcome with sleep – but it didn't seem to matter. The outside world was becoming softer and quieter. I was aware only of my big panting dog.

Then it happened. My head slumped on my chest and the next thing I became aware of was a loud graunching noise and a thump as my car mounted the concrete median strip. At the same moment Bella did her wind-the-window-down trick again and the air rushed in at me from all angles. Dazed and confused, I glanced up to see oncoming traffic. It looked evil and menacing; I knew I had to step on the brake. My foot was searching for the pedal, but somehow it couldn't or wouldn't do what I was telling it to, and it just floated above it. Seconds passed, horrifically scary, until my foot finally connected with the pedal – the correct pedal – and the car stopped. Other motorists were sounding their horns. I was saved from further humiliation because the traffic in my lane had halted in order to turn right.

This wait gave me precious time to gather myself. I was absolutely terrified, heart racing, mouth dry, brain fogged. I knew I must get home, and home was across this busy intersection with heavy five o'clock traffic driving at me. I don't know how I did that next bit. It felt like dicing with death, but eventually it was my turn at the front of the queue, there was a break in the traffic and away I went. Once on the Halswell stretch I found myself travelling at around forty kilometres per hour, but at least I was heading in the right direction – towards the hills and home. I don't recall much of that journey except that I stuck to my slow speed and that eventually I found myself coming into Governors Bay.

I turned left at the bottom of the hill, back towards Lyttelton, then into our drive – a right turn, down and into the carport. Relief. I tried to undo Bella's leash so that she could leave the car but this task proved almost impossible. Saliva, dog breath – then she was free, bounding and jumping. Freaking out completely, I made my way to the house. A bath, yes, that's what I needed. I was tired and it would revive me. But I should ring the medical centre and let them know. My doctor had said that if there were any changes I must ring her. I would ask the medical centre to call her at home. She would know what to do.

I rang the medical centre – the advice was to come straight in. I couldn't drive, of course. Philip wasn't due back for a further twenty minutes or more, then it would take another fifteen or twenty for us to reach the medical centre. They would be closed by then, and no, they wouldn't wait. They said my own doctor wasn't answering her mobile.

In the middle of all this I realised I had missed my appointment at the medical school. When I rang my colleague I was too embarrassed to tell him the real reason I hadn't turned up. Mark called in from Auckland on the other line while I was trying to explain myself. I was deceiving myself, telling them both that I was fine.

Then the medical centre rang back: I must go to Accident and Emergency at the hospital. Okay, I thought, I'll get Philip to take me there. I was embarrassed about asking him, however, knowing that, like me, he would be tired and hungry. When I asked the medical centre if A & E would know who I was and what it was about, they assured me that they would ring the hospital and explain.

Eight

I left home with Philip at around 7 PM after struggling with a skirt zip, which he finally had to do up. I can still recall the horrible feeling of the complete lack of strength in my left hand, and the desperate, black hopelessness that almost overcame me on the way into town.

'Do you ever really worry about the future?' I asked Philip. 'I feel I have no future. I want to give up. Things are too hard.'

'What you need,' said Philip, 'is a treat.' I was grateful for his attempt to cheer me up.

When I presented myself at A & E the woman behind the reception grille looked at me quizzically. No, there had been no communication from the medical centre about my arrival. No, they had no access to the fax sent by my doctor to the neurological clinic two days before. The clinic was closed for the day. The wait would be a few hours. I explained that I was in extreme need of food. Would it be okay if my friend took me off to eat, after which we would return? She looked at me very oddly, obviously completely disbelieving that anything was the matter with me. 'Well, if you leave, you'll slip off the computer. It might take you a long time to get back in the queue.' I heard myself say that I would take my chances. I was just too hungry.

Philip rang a favourite restaurant in town. It seemed slightly ridiculous to be making such a brief visit to a place where I usually sat for hours savouring my food, but I wasn't saying no. The food was gratefully received and it made me feel better, as did the lovely comforting environment, the care and the conversation. I tired very quickly and was reminded I must go back to A & E.

It was weird, but I felt kind of fraudulent being there and involving Philip. So I asked him to wait in the car and said I would let him know by mobile what was happening. It was now about 9.30 PM. I reported that I was back to waiting and more waiting. I tried to contact Lutz, my medical school colleague inside the hospital. He was still on a meal break, but eventually we caught up and tried to have a bit of a work meeting sitting there in the ghastliness of A & E, with the Madrid train bombings on the TV screen near us.

Ben, a friend's son, had rung me from Madrid during the day. He was very distressed and needed to talk. His mother wasn't answering so he'd phoned me. I was vague, not my usual self at all. Poor Ben, I had let him down. I don't know why I didn't contact my son Ollie − probably because I was trying not to worry him or disturb his last few days with his girlfriend.

At last I was called in. By now Philip was snoozing in the car outside. At 11.30 PM or so I was in a cubicle in A & E, which seemed deserted. I saw the occasional person, but otherwise it was empty. I felt so alone. I rang Philip and told him to go home − I would get a cab and contact him if I needed to.

A delightful young man finally shows up, picks up my clipboard − empty to date − and asks me the first question, pen poised. Then his beeper goes. 'Oh, I'm sorry, I have to go, they need me.' And that's it, he's swallowed up, gone. No other staff appear. Oh, there's the cleaner: she comes by a few times and wipes the lights opposite me. I begin sitting on a chair with a pillow leaning against a wall. Now I'm unashamedly lying on the bed, drifting in and out of a strange sleep. My medical school colleague makes his last visit for the night. He's going home.

My intern finally returns, hugely apologetic. He does some

quick neurological tests, one of which I fail dismally, my left hand dropping away significantly. I'm so spaced out I don't care much about anything. He comments that 'something is going on' and heads off with his recommendation to the neurological registrars. I don't know what happens then, but instead of taking me off for a scan the intern comes back and says that right now I should go home; someone will contact me in the morning to bring me back for a scan.

Okay, okay, so I must get back to Governors Bay. It's 1.30 AM. I return to the ghastly waiting area. The battery in my mobile is flat. I go to the public taxi telephone and dial. By the time the taxi arrives I feel drunk with tiredness and pain. I try to get into the car and then I smell it – cigarette smoke. 'Look,' I explain to the driver, 'no offence to you but someone's been smoking in your cab and I feel ill and I can't travel for half an hour in this smoky environment.' He protests but I know I can't stay in that car, so I step out, say goodbye and start the process again. Another cab arrives, this time smoke-free, and off we go.

In retrospect, of course, I was so ill I should have taken up Philip's earlier invitation to stay at his house. But my own bed seemed inviting and in the morning there would be animals to feed. It was 2 AM or so before we reached Governors Bay. I should have asked the driver to wait while I got into the house, but I no longer had clear judgement and my decisions were becoming fairly random. Life was something I was struggling through, becoming more and more a stranger to it. Assuring the taxi driver that I was okay, I moved unsteadily away down the path to the house and made it inside.

I can remember little about the rest of the night expect that I didn't sleep much. I sat in bed propped up by pillows. By this stage I liked to keep a light on at night because I felt so uncertain and couldn't cope with the dark. I noted a cup and saucer dropped on the stairs: I must have tried to make a cup of tea.

And then it was the morning of the 12th, and I realised that in all my confusion I had forgotten to send a present to my darling grandson Arlo in Australia, whose birthday it was.

Nine

I woke from my fitful sleep early on March the 12th, but I can't remember anything until Lavinia, my housekeeper, arrived. Fortunately, for some reason that week dear Lavinia, who always cleans on a Thursday, was coming on Friday. She is totally deaf in one ear and partially deaf in the other, so communications don't always flow easily. This morning was one of those times. Another symptom of my condition was that my voice was becoming less and less strong. Mark had been commenting on this but I had no energy to project it. I tried to call out to Lavinia but she just went on with her work – I could hear her cheerful whistling as she shuffled in her slippers to the sink.

It wasn't until Ollie and Philip arrived that something started to happen in my favour. I'd been ringing the medical centre since 8.30 AM – first I was put on hold, then told that someone would get back to me. Finally, on my third try, I'd persisted and got someone to talk to me. It all seemed like a nightmare. My doctor wasn't in that day and she hadn't cleared her mobile messages so didn't know that anything else had happened to me. But she'd definitely said that if I hadn't been contacted by the hospital for a scan by Thursday – the previous day – I must contact her again.

Even trying to push the buttons on the phone was such an effort that I almost gave up. Then the medical centre staff rang back and said I had an appointment to see a neurologist the following Tuesday. But what had happened to the fax my doctor had sent on the

9th, and the notes from the doctor in A & E last night requesting an immediate scan? The system appeared to be breaking down horribly and yet I just didn't seem to care any more. My usual indignation in such circumstances had gone out the window.

I remember, in the middle of all this, getting out of bed and struggling to the dressing table in order to put on some lipstick. I knew I looked pretty ghastly, and I had to remedy that. It must have been a bizarre sight – my pale face decorated with red lippy. I remember my dearest Ollie coming in, sitting on my bed and asking me what was happening. Then Philip arrived, very concerned. He went off to work – 'Ring me if you need me. Sarah will be back later today and she'll be in touch.' And then Ollie took over. 'Mum, you have to get a scan today.' I knew he was right.

But now, about noon, the phone rang and it was my doctor. Deciding to drop by the medical centre, she had noticed that my notes were out and saw I'd rung in. She talked to me and to Ollie. Arrangements would be made a short while later. They were. Ollie said he would go home to his place fifteen minutes away, get changed and then take me for a scan at a private hospital. I didn't care. Lavinia, by now fully aware and concerned, brought me tea and helped me to get showered and dressed. This part is all so blurred in my memory. I know this, though: I still wore my 'uniform'. No buttons, no zips, no difficult decisions to make about what went with what. Disintegration complete.

My next memory is of arriving at St George's Hospital with Ollie. My head was heavy and uncomfortable. I hated lying down on the narrow bed for the scan and seeing the technician standing over me – 'Don't get up, please stay still.' Then another person, male, interpreted the scan result and Ollie's pale, anxious face appeared above me. I had it explained to me that there was a bleed – a significant bleed. My worst fears were confirmed. No, not my worst – that would have been an inoperable tumour. This bleed was something I'd never even thought of.

I lay in a very pleasant room at St George's. Ollie, beside me, was keeping very calm, although he was extremely distressed. And then a consultant explained to me that I must go the public hospital for surgery. Not immediately, he assured me, noting my rising panic. 'They'll observe and assess you, and maybe in a few days they'll operate and drain the blood – something like that. You can go with your son – it'll be quicker than an ambulance.' Ollie brought his car round, but I can recall nothing of the trip.

Ten

We're at the door of A & E – we have the scans, we'd been told we'd be expected. Ollie must park the car. I'm standing, very unsteady. The doors open. I head for the nearest seat. Like the night before, the TV is blaring forth, with bad static, an update on the Madrid train bombing. I start gradually to fall to the left. No one is there to notice and I don't care, and then there's Ollie at the reception desk. 'My mother's brain is bleeding. Get her a bed.' Quiet but definite. At last someone is going to do something.

Memory: the neurological registrar appears, his face without emotion. Get on with it, I'm thinking. And then there's Mark. He's arrived from somewhere, an airport I imagine, and is trying to get assurances from the registrar. Ollie, calm but stressed, is leading the proceedings.

Memory: a room for children, its decorations suggest. Comings and goings, curtains swinging, the ugliness of A & E. By now it's around 3 or 4 PM. People are hovering. There's an air of waiting, of expectation. I don't know it yet, but at this point Maxine, who will become a good friend, is in theatre undergoing delicate neurological surgery with the medical team who will soon operate on me.

Memory: in the neurological ward and my dear friend Sarah has arrived. She's rubbing my feet. Someone is washing my hair. My hair was washed yesterday. I wonder what shampoo they're using – I'm so fussy about the brand I use. And now someone is talking about cutting off my top with scissors. 'Hang on a minute,' I hear myself say, 'this top was bought in Paris last year. You most definitely will not cut it.' Amused, startled – I don't know what the reaction is, but I think I hear Sarah supporting me and then the garment is gently rolled up over my head.

Memory: the surgeon, holding a skull that has a detachable top. It is smooth, dark brown and small. He is also holding a drill – a small hand drill. He tells me that he will be drilling two holes in my skull so that the blood can be drained. The hair will be shaved in two small areas. It all sounds pretty simple really.

The part that scares me most is the anaesthetic – any drug-taking in fact. Having never had a general anaesthetic and having suffered from anaphylactic shock on at least two occasions (evidently I'm allergic to the additives in local anaesthetics), along with having a myriad of drug sensitivities, I'm not a great candidate. There's a lot of discussion and assurances that any drug will be administered slowly and nothing will be used that isn't absolutely necessary. It's a totally terrifying experience for me, the control freak, to give myself over to medics.

At the end of my bed are Sarah and Philip, and beside me are Mark and Ollie. Various nursing staff come and go, fairly faceless and nameless, except for Jeanette, who has a warm, comforting smile; she is my protector, my go-between. And then Lutz's face appears around the curtain: 'Good luck, Rosie. I know it will go well.'

Mark is talking a lot to Sarah about the history of the Chathams. I can hear his voice going on above me – houses, history, Maori history, landscapes. Sarah isn't saying much; Mark is giving what seems to be a lecture, trying to distract himself. How bizarre – these are to be my last conscious memories for a while, the history of the Chathams, and I'm not in the slightest bit interested. Then I see Mark start to open the brown paper bag he has in his hand. It crackles and out comes a large panini. I feel terribly sick – the smell, the sight of it. 'Oh please Mark,' I say, 'not here.'

'Sorry, I'll go outside to eat it.'

He leaves. Then the orderly arrives and Mark has to be located. I'm not impressed: he still smells of panini.

Mark and Ollie are beside me. The anaesthetist is reassuring me, and then I'm on my way, through the door, down towards the operating table and the huge overhead lights. The anaesthetist tries a little of the anaesthetic in my lure. I'm okay and then I'm not there…

Eleven

The first thing I remember after the operation is the surgeon saying, with his thumbs up, 'Struck oil.' And then pain, pain, and an unbelievable acid stomach and shaking. There were other patients around me; I could hear moaning, but most people were very sedated. For me, with my allergies, there was only good old Panadol. I wanted my husband.

I needed the comfort of human touch. 'Please, nurse, please can you touch me – hold me for a minute?' I begged through chattering teeth. She looked startled. This clearly wasn't something she regarded as a reasonable request – we were in recovery, after all – and she moved away. I felt as though I were in a morgue. I was totally awake by now, unable to move. All around me were the humps of bodies on beds or cots.

I arrived in the special care unit in Ward 28 and Mark was waiting there for me. I begged him to get me some relief for my acid stomach and some sparkling water. He went, and I waited and waited. I thought it was midnight or 1 AM, and then I must have slept because when I next woke there was the water but no Mark. He had been and gone. The night was so long. I couldn't move but my hearing was acute. I could only see straight ahead of me. Opposite me was a woman with a turban bandage and a wet cloth over her face. Occasionally she moved a little.

The night was interspersed every few minutes by observations, or obs. A nurse shone a torch in my eyes and asked me questions:

What year is it? What day is it? Who is the Prime Minister? Then she checked my blood pressure, heart rate and temperature. I could hear the answers of the woman opposite – she sounded so tired, so very ill – but I don't remember hearing my own answers.

During that first night, March the 13th, I began the humbling journey of being a patient, vulnerable to my caregivers, on the receiving end of our public health system and all its peculiarities. But I was alive, thanks to the skills of my neurosurgeon and his dedicated team. I was, as he put it, the recipient of a very simple head operation, one he could do with his eyes closed. Oh yes? The ward was full of people with the most extraordinarily complex head ailments. What a macabre lot we were.

As I lay there, the sense most heightened for me was hearing. The sounds of the room seemed incredibly loud: the monitors bleeping, clicking and going off when something disturbed their rhythm; the various breathing noises and the mutterings of delirium; the voice of an ebullient nurse talking to a nearby patient, then resuming her conversation with a colleague about how she couldn't wait for the shift to be over. I found any noise, any movement, exhausting. I couldn't understand this nurse. She seemed oblivious to all four of us. Did she think that her bounce and booming talk were going to cheer us up?

It must have been around 6 AM when someone said, 'Hello, you've got a lovely voice.' So I said, 'Thank you. So have you.' And she did: it was gentle and cultivated. It was Maxine, the woman with the turban opposite me. Perhaps I had one of those too – that didn't even occur to me. Although we were too ill then to talk, we had made a connection that was to remain. We were like two hurt birds, knocked down, unable to rise. It was at this time that the shift changed – always a welcome event, I came to realise. With the changeover came dawn and the hope of a new day – the first of my new life.

Twelve

Memory: when the bandage was taken off on that first day I felt a rush of cool air on my head. My thoughts weren't jumbled and my left hand worked – yes, it passed the finger test, the Rosie indicator. Wow, I thought, I'm fixed. Yes, I feel as though a bus has knocked me down, and my back and neck and head feel as if they have sustained some massive rugby-type injury, but I'm not dead, the blood has been drained, I'll be bouncing soon.

The man selling newspapers came in – '*Press, Press,*' he called, as he passed among beds whose occupants weren't able to acknowledge him. 'Yes, I'll have one,' I said. But I had to pay money, and where would that be? What and where were my personal possessions? My bed had been cranked up a little so I could try to look at the paper. A quick look, then exhaustion.

Memory: touching my head. There was no hair – just the weird feeling of my bare skull. An unappetising breakfast arrived. After the medical entourage left I waited for Mark. I, of course, was looking forward to him bringing something feminine for me to wear – something to replace the hospital-issue winceyette PJs – and something to clean my teeth with. But no. When Mark arrived he stared at me, trying to take in my new look, I suppose. He then put down a book. What was it? *On Call*, a textbook containing medical emergencies likely to be encountered by a doctor on duty. It was part of the pack of information I had been given to prepare me for my teaching role at the medical school. I had been studying these scenarios, trying to gather ideas when preparing my classes, so this book had been sitting beside the bed. It was not, however, quite what I would have chosen for a person who had just undergone brain surgery. And where was the silk nightie or the toothpaste and toothbrush? Ah well, he'd forgotten them.

I was shifted to a ward room – a dark corner. At that stage I didn't care. I felt a little better when flowers and messages began to arrive, but the anger and grief wouldn't go away. How could my husband of thirty-three years, who professed to love me, have stood by and watched my decline and not been more concerned? I wanted someone to blame.

I think he was scared – the arrogance and rudeness were masking the real feelings underneath. My dear son Ollie, who had been my primary support person through the past three days, was showing the effects of the trauma. Forgive your parents, I wanted to say to him, that you've had to wear so much responsibility.

So there I was in the neuro unit, sitting in bed with not two holes, as promised, but three drilled in my head. The bleed had evidently been wider than estimated from the scan, necessitating an extra hole. I was as bald as a baby on one side of my head. But I could use my left side again; I could see, think, remember. I was so lucky. But my emotions were raw. My head was cold. I'd had to give up being in control. I'd had to put my faith in a team of strangers. What had happened to me?

The scan taken at St George's on March the 12th 2004 showed that I had a large blood clot, or haematoma, over the surface of the brain, causing a ten-millimetre mid-line shift from right to left. It was this brain shift that had caused such major problems to my everyday living.

Epidural or subdural haematomas can develop suddenly from a severe head injury, or they can also develop slowly after a relatively minor injury. Mine was the latter: the bleeding had occurred over a number of weeks, leaking into the space between the dura (the tough outer layer of the brain that is attached to the inner surface of the skull) and the brain. As the subdural haematoma increased in size, it began to compress my brain. Surgical removal of the blood was required quickly. Without intervention the bleeding would cause death.

The clot was removed by drilling three burr holes in the skull and draining it. A right frontal and two parietal burr holes allowed the drainage of the haematoma.

15 MARCH. *Sick stomach, legs numb, saliva drying – panic attack 12.30 AM. Fear – terrible fear. Night staff problems.*

16 MARCH. *I'm walking with assistance. I'm stunned by what has happened to me.*

18 MARCH. *Surrounded by loving gestures from friends and family. And although it looks like expressions of sympathy for a funeral, I'm not dead. I'm getting a chance to experience the loving from people while I'm alive to enjoy it. My head hurts, my right ear feels a bit deaf and very sore. I'm feeling faint. Every day has so many moods to it. My neck and upper shoulder are so bruised – what caused that? The nights are so long. I so much want to get better in a hurry now and this is obviously not going to be happening. Nurses and doctors keep telling me, 'It's not a broken arm or leg – it's your brain, your head. It needs time, lots of time.'*

Thirteen

Distraction was the key to getting through those early days and nights – and Panadol, of course. And it was very important for me to continue trying to be feminine despite the hairstyle, despite the face obviously alarmed by its new circumstances, the black rings under the eyes and the pallor.

19 MARCH. *My hairstylist comes to the hospital. I've showered and my hair is washed. I trust him. He's amazing, unfazed by my mauled hairdo. He sets to, to save what he can and give the illusion of hair where there's none. He does well – I'm amazed and pleased, and he doesn't even charge me!*

20 MARCH. *I'm home and I can handle the stairs. That's lucky because the only bathroom is halfway between the bedroom on the top floor and the living areas on the ground floor.*

21 MARCH. *Improvements. First walk to the vegetable garden with Mark and to the little summerhouse in the garden – walking is slow and awkward, but I am walking. I watch Mark pick beautiful tomatoes. The autumn harvest is beginning.*

22 MARCH. *Slept much better in own bed. Walked with assistance a circuit of the garden. Afternoon – walked with Mark to the Scout Den, a distance of 300 m. Felt the sea breeze on my hair. Delicious feeling.*

Afternoon rest followed by strange feelings. The worst sensations are numbness and pain on the side of my head, stiff face, closing of right eye, pressure sensations on side of head, faintness. What have they done to me? The best sensations – more clarity, vision improving, ability to have true rest improving.

I had a phone call from the counsellor at my doctor's surgery. 'I've been asked to offer you some free counselling sessions,' she said.

'Oh,' I replied, 'counselling on what?'

'On your near-death experience,' she said. 'I do trauma counselling.'

'Well,' I said, 'I don't think I want that right now. I'm enjoying being alive. Now, if you're offering counselling on my inability to help with my husband's business, that's another matter.'

She agreed to my suggestion and an appointment was made for April the 6th.

24 MARCH. *This is day 12 after the operation. I'm doing quite well.*

1 APRIL. *Feeling very ill – faint. The accountant visits to discuss business. I can't cope. After two hours, I've collapsed. Feel so bad. My doctor turns up to visit me at home. She's concerned. She brings the date for the scan forward.*

2 APRIL. *A day from hell. A visit to the hospital. The scan shows a new bleed and I'm told I must have another surgical procedure. It's the only way. This is too much. I'll run away. I can't go through that pain again. Can't let them go back into those delicate wounds. Oh my God...*

On the eighth day after the operation a scan had confirmed a significant reduction in the size of the haematoma. However, in ten to fifteen per cent of cases like mine, a re-accumulation can occur; I was one of these unlucky ones. The scan now showed that the haematoma had two densities: an outer higher density and an inner lower density, suggesting an intermediate membrane, which proved to be the case.

I asked if I could have an hour outside the hospital. Mark drove me to the gates of the gardens and helped me to a warm spot under a tree. I was hungry. He said he would buy me food – some pasta from a local café. And so I sat, trying to grasp what I'd just been told. I'll run away, I thought, but then reality sank in. Where? How? I can't fly anywhere – instant death. I wept, and then I ate, savouring the flavours of lemon and chicken and pasta, the warmth of the sun on my skin, and the dryness of the pine needles, a cushion under me.

My poor family. How difficult for them. Well, I'll just have to cope. I've coped once, and I'll have to cope again. Added to my bad news was that of Mark's work situation. A possible new client wasn't coming on board and our main client had decided to pull out, with no thanks and no recognition of my situation or Mark's distress about it. The mercilessness of big business hit us hard that day. We were bewildered by our losses.

The family gathered their energies. I was allowed home for the weekend. The next surgical intervention would be on Tuesday, April the 6th: no counselling after all. My daughter, Aimee, was on her way from Townsville, arriving at midnight on Saturday.

The weekend went by in a blur of loving embraces from family and friends. Seattle friends made a surprise visit on Saturday lunchtime, and I managed to set a table on the veranda of the little house. Then my darling Aimee arrived, bringing protection, flowers, food and laughter. I made a video clip with Ollie and Aimee. My head was full of pressure but I was calm.

On April the 5th – a grey, cold, wintry day – I returned to hospital, to wait. Visits from friends filled in the time. The anaesthetist came by, a different one this time. I could feel the anxiety kicking in – would he do what was done before? Could I relax in this knowledge?

6 APRIL. *What does one do to fill in time while waiting for a brain operation? Listen to the ducks quacking on the river below? Tune in to the banter on the ward? File your nails and put on lipstick? Or just sit or lie and wait. It's like a plane trip to a faraway place, sitting in the uncomfortable part of economy. Some bad weather patches are predicted en route.*

Fourteen

I awoke from my second procedure feeling totally disgusting, much worse than I could ever remember feeling in my life. I couldn't move my head at all without the world spinning, and tubes coming out of me in all directions made this impossible anyhow. I can't remember much of that first day. Aimee tells me she was there. I think my friend Sarah came, and Mark of course. When Aimee went home for a rest, Mark slept for a while in the dayroom while Sarah sat with me. I never want to feel that bad again. It horrifies me to remember it. I just wanted Aimee, Mark or Sarah to stay with me, to be close. I felt so vulnerable, especially among the night nursing staff with whom I had been so unimpressed during my previous visit.

The second surgery had required re-entry to two of the burr holes, and the opening of the outer subdural space to a depth of one-and-a-half centimetres to reach the intermediate membrane. This had been opened and forceps used to gain access to the smaller, deeper haematoma.

The same process had been carried out with the frontal burr hole, again using forceps to drain the subdural fluid, which this time was described as 'a little dark brown and tarry'. The subdural spaces had then been irrigated with warm saline, so my brain had been given a spring clean. Wow, I was fortunate.

I was back in the intensive care room of the neurological ward. It was the same scenario, only this time everything was different.

I'd been comforting myself beforehand by rationalising that as I knew what had happened last time and how I had felt, this would surely be an advantage second time around. But no. Of course, the sensation of dependence, the heightened emotions, the smells and sounds of the ward, the nurses and the consultants were all familiar. What was different was my feeling of helplessness and hopelessness. I was more tearful, less able to move, more frightened. I tried to repeat the patterns to my day that had comforted me the first time, but that didn't always work.

Opposite me this time was Nev the builder. God knows what had happened to him. He looked all right, but was bandaged in the usual turban style that was the speciality of our ward. Nev was erratic in his answering of the questions put to him, sometimes wandering right off track, causing the nurse on duty to persist more loudly and more often. 'Come on, Nev, what day is it? Where are you?' One night the phone rang at about 11 PM. 'Oh Nev, it's your mum. Here, you can speak to her if you like.' Nev moved slightly in the bed and the nurse put the phone against the bandage where his ear should be. 'Yeah Mum, I'm okay, yeah, yeah, sure Mum,' he shouted.

The call over, Nev began one of many severely disturbed nights. Delirium took over. 'Oi, Nige… Watch out, Nige, watch that kitchen joinery. Bring me a ratchet, no, bring me the spanner. Now, yeah, I said I need it now. Hey, watch it mate, watch out.' This monologue from Nev would go on and on. Just before dawn he went quiet. When the staff nurse came to test him, she couldn't get a sound out of him. He's dead, I thought. She shouted, standing over him, 'Come on Nev, what day is it?' He finally gave an answer of sorts, then seemed to go quiet again until breakfast arrived.

I had had a terrible night. I felt unbelievably bad, but I had survived with my marbles intact – or so it seemed. I was lucky. I looked at the breakfast they had delivered. I should eat something, but how? I would just watch Nev. I couldn't believe it: Nev, who had seemed so precariously ill all night, was delivered breakfast on a bed tray. The back of his bed was cranked up. They tapped him, and he opened his eyes. They put a spoon out for him. He picked it up and began to shovel in the cold porridge. When he came to the end he picked up the plastic bowl, brought it to his lips and sucked out the last remaining bits of porridge and milk. It's amazing what the human body can achieve, I thought, as I struggled even to move my head from centre to left or right. The vertigo was debilitating.

At some point my surgeon stood at the foot of the bed and said, 'Well, that was a success. Get up and have a run if you feel like it!' His joke was so far from reality that it found no resonance with me.

Fifteen

So I was fixed again, was I? What did that actually mean in terms of what I could or could not do? Looking back now, I wonder if it would have been useful at that point to have been given a more realistic time frame for my recovery. Or was the doctors' method the right one – just letting me go a few days ahead, rather than knowing I had months or even years of rehabilitation in front of me? If I met a friend in my situation I think I would tell him or her to expect the unexpected, to be ready for surprises and unusual symptoms, and to block out social and work calendars for at least six months. I didn't do this, and so often felt such a failure because I just couldn't seem to get going again.

So the recovery process began. As before, I had run the gauntlet of medical staff, hospital procedures and post-operative intensive care, and now I was on my own again, trying to piece together a disrupted life. Once more the room filled with flowers and cards. I had brought back to hospital some of my favourite cards from three weeks before, along with my vases and homeopathic remedies. I had my bed by the window: the best therapy was to watch the skyscape and, during the day, the beauty of the gardens below.

It was colder now, late autumn. The clothes my visitors wore began to reflect this. It was Easter and, true to new hospital policy, the patients were being shipped out and off for the long weekend. No hospital-issue hot cross buns for them. I was in a large room with enough beds for five people, but there were only two others and they were due to go home at Easter. I didn't care. More peace for me.

Aimee, my dear supportive daughter, had to leave to get back to her two children and husband in Townsville. He had to return to his geology work and there was no one to mind the children. I hated to see her go. My son Mischa was coming to visit, as was my sister Angie, whom I hadn't seen for months. Phone calls began coming in again from loving friends and family far away. But speaking on the phone was a trial – I would talk briefly, then say I couldn't manage any more. Yes, it hurt my head but, more than that, it took up too much energy – energy I needed to sustain myself through the next minutes and hours in this weird new life.

Not being able to walk at first was a shock. Why couldn't I? There was nothing wrong with my legs. A big achievement after that second operation was when I walked, or rather shuffled, half a circuit of the ward. Some days I found I could walk a bit more.

One day Mischa took me out in the wheelchair to the café on the river below. I slid onto a real chair and had a cup of tea and a scone. The change of scene was wonderful. Looking straight ahead was very important, as side-to-side views incurred stress and giddiness. There was also a trip in the wheelchair, rugged up against the cold, around the park, with my son Ollie and my sister as escorts. Taking photos from wheelchair height was a new experience – some good shots resulted.

Everything looked new to me, and marvellous. I had never really looked at the world like this before.

Sixteen

Lying down flat in a quiet environment was essential for many hours each day. When I was awake, my powers of observation were still acute. Human beings and their behaviour continued to intrigue me.

My new room-mate was a kindly woman called Flora. She was illiterate, eking out a livelihood in a small coastal town, where she survived on a benefit. She had suffered a tumour, and I felt for her as she recounted to me the year before her surgery and diagnosis, knowing too well her depression and feelings of inadequacy as she struggled with her increasingly useless body. The strangeness of our circumstances shocked me as I lay there. Here we were, so utterly different in our backgrounds and our expectations of life, yet similarly flattened by our surgeries. I felt embarrassed about my mass of floral arrangements and my deliveries of delicious food, my visitors and their offerings, my children, my husband.

It was the day before Flora's departure when she told me part of her life story.

'Men, you know, we can do without them. I like my daughter, she's so good to me, but men, well I think I'm over them. One day about ten years ago I was standing in the shower when it came to me like a flash of light: "You don't need him in your life any more. You need to ask him to leave." So I did. "Look," I said, "I've had enough, I want you to leave. You can have the boys and I'll keep the girl." And so he did, carrying on with his gambling and laying about. I still saw the boys. They didn't move far away.

'Anyway my ex got bored, so he got himself a Filipino bride. She was young, wanted babies. He had a problem there though, because he'd been fixed, you know. The boys were getting older, and he had the idea to ask the oldest to help out – help his dad – so he did, and they got the baby. That one's about four now and there's another one too. I don't really have anything to do with them. Dear little things, though. The problem now is that the Filipino wife wants to go home to live, back to the Philippines with the kids. But she doesn't want my ex – she's in love, she says, with my boy. Yeah, but he's married already. Bit of a mess.'

I was stunned by what she'd told me and managed only a short response. 'Do the locals know?' I asked.

'Oh, yeah, they know.'

Anyway, Flora couldn't wait to be back in her house and to be a granny again to her daughter's little child and the other one on the way. Despite having so little, she was happy with her lot and happy to be alive. So she went – out into a freezing day by ambulance, ill equipped with clothing but well equipped with attitude.

The hospital days passed by as they do, demarcated by the military precision of meals and visiting times and doctors' visits, and the long, long nights of sleeplessness. The waiting to get better.

Memory: one morning at about 3 AM I felt a weight on my bed and looked up to see an elderly addled man trying to climb in. I managed to muster an indignant 'What are you doing?' and 'Which ward do you think you're in?' I discovered he was from a ward below. On a trip to the toilet, he had shuffled his way into the lift and stepped off onto the wrong floor. He shuffled off with muttered apologies into the endless corridors.

I remember, too, an elderly woman, Ellen, overwhelmed and consumed by grief, sobbing relentlessly, calling to me from a neighbouring bed, disturbed by the nursing chatter of the midnight shift. Grieving for her losses, she wanted mostly to be left alone.

I recall, too, a tattooed guy with one ear torn off and now sewed back on. Pale and shaky, with black circles under his eyes, he was shuffling and dazed like the rest of us. His wounds were the result of a car crash in which he had been pushed off the road and left there bleeding for hours. We spoke occasionally. He didn't sound anything like the tough image he would have portrayed out there in his other life. Would he grieve for his losses?

And then there was the bird lady, Alma. Feathered visitors – pigeons and seagulls – would land on our window ledge, opportunists waiting for the chance of food. Alma would relish their visits. Early each morning she would take from her locker all the bread crusts and uneaten sandwiches from the day before. Then, swinging her short legs over the bed into the waiting lounge slippers, she would begin her shuffle to the window, cooing and calling to the birds – 'Come on my little beauties, come on' – her speech muffled by a lack of teeth, stitches in her mouth and a strong European accent. She would push up the window and decorate the sills with her offerings. There would be a few moments of feathers and flutter and beaks and general chaos as the pecking order was established, and then quiet – and all the food would be gone. One day Alma opened the window a little more than usual and put the sandwich crusts inside on the sill, and two or three pigeons walked in. They were our room-mates for a short while that morning, much to our delight.

Alma would stand, her back to us, just gazing from the window, saying over and over, 'I want to go home, I want to go home, I want to go home.'

Seventeen

I craved a bath – with lavender and candles. Why was there no bath tub in this ward? It seemed ludicrous that the comfort of hot water and healing aromas weren't available for such sick people as us. A tub visit was organised for me, and I was wheeled downstairs to occupational therapy. I was so grateful to the therapist who organised this. The bath wasn't very pretty but the water was deliciously hot. How wonderful it was to slip into that scented warmth, lying there supported and taking in the lavender aromas, resting and dreaming for a brief while away from the ward. Those visits to the bath tub were an important step in my early recovery, even if I did feel extremely faint afterwards. It was better than shuffling on the Zimmer frame to the ugly shower units in the ward.

My visitors were always a comfort – those lovely people who came, making the effort in their busy lives to see me in this place. I loved looking at what they wore, feeling the outside world come in to me, touching the warmth of their skin on the balmy autumnal days. Details of faces, voices, adornments became my companions.

I couldn't read. The nurses had said, 'Look at the magazines, but you probably won't be able to read.' That seemed ridiculous but, to my amazement, it was true. My eyesight had changed anyway – looking through my old glasses was a huge strain – but it wasn't just the need for new, stronger glasses. Somehow I couldn't cope with – nor did I want to cope with – the complexity of reading in anything but short bursts. Wonderful magazines began to arrive with friends. I lay and fantasised about walking on beaches in the Seychelles or staying in magnificent luxury in the Maldives. I remembered pieces of my life. How lucky I was to have had so many adventures to colour my new lonely existence: the lunches in the Luberon in southeast France, watching wild game from a fenced compound in South Africa, drifting in clear blue water off the coast of Turkey…

And then there were the recipe magazines – those culinary journeys filled in many hours and began to excite my taste buds. I knew I needed to eat, and also that I needed to want to eat. I couldn't cope with the hospital food and I was very fortunate that family and friends kept up a shuttle service between local restaurants and my ward. A chicken green curry, with coconut cream and coriander – an old favourite from a local Thai restaurant – arrived, as did a tasty beetroot salad from Sarah's kitchen and organic yogurts and fresh fruit gathered by Mark. There were hot chicken salads for lunches, home-made biscuits for morning and afternoon teas, plenty of sparkling mineral water, a lemon- and olive-flavoured pasta made by Mischa. Mark had delivered some of my pretty china dishes early on, and to see food in these was a real pleasure. I surrounded myself in a cocoon of beauty: flowers, drawings pinned on the walls from my siser-in-law, Robyn, cards from my lovely grandchildren, scarves and ribbons on the bed ends, books and magazines.

An alternative therapist called Eva brought her gift of healing in the form of homeopathic and Bach flower remedies: arnica drops and ointment for the bruising on my neck and back; and Rescue Remedy drops and Rescue Cream for the shock. Through these remedies and massage, she helped put the pieces back together and calmed me from the inside out. The medical staff were very supportive about our alternative treatments. Foot massage was an important first step towards being touched; it also allowed me to 'let go' briefly. One of the things I noticed after such major surgery was that I did not feel safe, either in myself or with others. I know this reaction would have slowed down my recovery had I not got those massages early on. I also felt I wanted other women around me: it was the comfort factor – as many women experience after childbirth.

Then it was time to go home, on Easter Sunday, April the 11th 2004, my younger son Ollie's twenty-fourth birthday. Late in the day, Lavinia had put loving touches to the house, warming it and placing flowers in the vases. Dinner was supplied by the local pub chef and Eva had made a birthday cake for Ollie. So, at the beginning of the dark and cold of late autumn/early winter I was housed in my small and lovely home, where I would stay, cushioned from the world, for many months to come.

This second homecoming did not have quite the joy of the first. There was fear, too. What if my behaviour had contributed to the second bleed? I was afraid of pushing myself at all. And so the weeks and months of recuperation began.

Eighteen

25 APRIL. *I think it's a Sunday. I've been testing my brain with reading French — vocabulary so appallingly lacking, probably not as a result of my brain surgery, just previous life laziness. Still enjoy mostly reading newspapers and magazines, which is easier than coping with a book. Days pass by — autumn is closing. My health improves each day. It's three weeks since my last operation and I am making good progress. Maybe in another month I will be feeling good.*

How optimistic was that?

It was only later, months down the track, when I started seeing rehab personnel and other specialists more regularly, that I learned that I was in fact doing well and that the symptoms and exhaustion I was experiencing were all within the 'normal' range. My Accident Compensation Corporation (ACC) manager throughout this time was amazing — so supportive and reassuring. And my various consultants all told me constantly that I was doing well. If this was doing well, I thought, what was doing badly?

The occupational therapists had been right when they told me to manage my days, my rest, my visitors and telephone calls. Arrogantly, I thought, Oh yes, I can do more than that, I'll show them. That attitude got me nowhere fast.

It was good for me to keep my home environment ticking over as it always had — clean, organised, flowers in the vases, good smells coming from the kitchen. Having home help from people who cared about me and who wanted me to get better was a huge bonus.

A pattern for the day developed and *if* I adhered to this, things were manageable. I could expect to sleep better at night, and to suffer from less head pain and pressure, less crankiness and fewer feelings of weakness and despair.

In April and May of that first year a good day went like this. I would wake around 6 AM, look at some books and then get up around 8 AM. I would perhaps make the odd telephone call, then slowly organise and eat breakfast, before going back to bed for another two hours or so. I would then shower and perhaps shuffle around the garden paths, sometimes unaided, sometimes with a walking stick or a helping arm.

At 11.30 AM, I would get lunch prepared, organise a helper and outline tasks. Lunch was at noon, and then I would rest again for up to two hours or more, often gazing at magazines, particularly food magazines. At 3 PM I would come downstairs and prepare an evening meal.

It really helped me to try new recipes and to get my helpers to be kitchen hands, peeling, scraping, beating, dishwashing and so on. Sarah had us around to her house at least once a week, and each time a special food treat was lovingly prepared and served. These five-minute car trips were my first forays into the outside world. I knew her house well and felt utterly safe with her and Philip. And she always managed to distract me and make me feel like an attractive woman. We talked clothes and food and children, and planned for future events.

The threat of losing part of our property because of financial difficulties loomed over us all like a black cloud. My way of coping was to plan an alternative future garden – just in case. Having a project to focus on helped me to keep mentally focused and balanced. Lying in bed, I dreamed and planned, delighting in looking at brochures and selecting bulb and rose orders.

Nineteen

Our financial situation did not improve, so we decided to put part of our land on the market. Those days were terrible, as I lay on the window-seat with my wounded head and watched the land agent showing people around my garden. How I hated that intrusion on my privacy. How terrified I was of making a wrong move, of signing something I shouldn't. But we didn't sign. I have weird memories of people making good offers, but these all involved doing awful things to our beautiful garden. I don't think the land agents had ever had to contend with such unwilling vendors.

We had stipulated that anyone who made an offer above a certain amount would need to attend an interview with us so we could ascertain their intentions and their suitability as future neighbours. We had also stipulated that no developers were to be considered. 'Highly irregular, highly irregular,' we were told. 'Ah, but it's our land and our future,' we said, 'and we only get one opportunity to vet this process.' Dozens were interested but perhaps only five came up with offers worthy of consideration.

We chose the veranda of the little house for the interview with one man and his partner. He seemed to have the attitude of a developer. He wouldn't look at me – the first bad sign. He then showed us a magazine picture of a huge concrete house, completely inappropriate for these surroundings. I cautiously asked him why he would want a house so large when there were just the two of them. 'Ah well,' he said, 'between us we have five grown-up children and we want each of them to have a room they can feel is theirs when they come to stay.'

I looked at Mark, then said, 'So this picture is your idea of a house you would like to build.'

'Yes, yes, but I want more land. Would you consider selling the other section or part of it? I need more space.'

Well, one thing the operation had done was reduce my tolerance of crap, as well as adding a definiteness to my responses – probably as a result of the frontal lobe being squashed by blood. Seeing that Mark wasn't going to answer in a hurry, I turned to this man and said, 'I think you're in the wrong place.' He looked surprised, the land agent troubled.

'Yes, the wrong place,' I repeated. I mentioned some alternative areas. 'That's where this house plan would be appropriate. Just imagine if I agreed to this type of dwelling here. How would the neighbours feel about it? We need to honour the land we are caretakers of. No, you're in the wrong place.'

His face, and that of his partner and the land agent, looked stunned. My husband remained impassive, although I could see he did not disagree. So, despite the pleas from the potential buyer's partner and her attempts to reassure me that she loved our style of house and would never let him have his fantasy, there was no deal. We politely gave them tea and they went on their way.

Somehow, despite the fog I was in, Mark and I managed to find alternatives to selling. We were inspired by a telephone call from an older, wise and caring friend, who said, 'You can't sell that bit of land – it's your crown jewels. We'll help you to hold onto it.' Then he added, 'How much do you need to do that?'

We didn't actually take him up on his offer of financial assistance, but it was this powerful support and optimism that led us to the conclusion that we'd had enough losses and needed to save the garden. At that point, many alternatives were tossed about. Our architect friend Simon, who had designed our home, started making plans for houses in the bottom garden. He was on a rescue mission. Maybe we could have a high-end B&B on the land. Maybe… maybe… We tried out lots of ideas, all of which exhausted me. Then we went back to the bank and to our loyal friend and business associate in Australia. Our colleague listened and advised and hung in there with us. The bank listened and hung in there with us. It was a tough year, but we got through it.

13 MAY. *Yesterday was Mark's and my thirty-fourth wedding anniversary. The end of the world as I knew it, and a new one is emerging.*

On 21 May it was my daughter-in-law Sol's birthday. She and my son were staying in Nelson, and since there was another family birthday there that week it seemed a chance to celebrate and see our grandchildren, so Mark and I planned to go up by car. I still couldn't consider flying an option. I also knew that at the speed I was able to travel – a maximum of forty to sixty kilometres per hour – the drive would be an arduous one for both of us, so I planned carefully.

Step one, the leg from Christchurch to Hanmer, usually took two hours, but at our speed and with stops it would take maybe four hours. When we got there we decided on a visit to the hot pools. This was a mistake: the extreme temperature change made me very faint. After minutes in the pool I had to be taken to the medical bay. My second mistake was trying to walk, with Mark's assistance, from the motel to the pool. It was perhaps only 200 metres, but that was too far. I collapsed completely, in tears.

25 MAY. *A backward step or two has left me nervous and depressed. Bad feelings in my head – eye playing up. Lots of crying. Using a walking stick helps.*

In retrospect, that trip eight weeks after the operation was too much. I thought I was doing so well during the shared meal with the family, but I was in bed for a week afterwards.

Twenty

13 JUNE. *Today has been a good day. Walked almost to the jetty and back. Went out in the boat. Mark rang. Picnicked in the weak winter sunlight. Gardening happening at home – it's going to be wonderful this spring. My symptoms still are giddiness almost all of the time, even lying still. Usual weird stuff. Occasional internal earthquakes, where I feel as though I am going to fall off my chair or fall over. Hardly any headaches any more. Feelings of getting out of control at times. I speed up too much. I find doing some small physical activities a good antidote. Also massage and hot water (bath or shower or hot tub). I have periods of intense fear that this state will never change. The best antidote is distraction. Good food, good video, good laugh – taking care not to laugh with too much energy or the head hurts. Worst thing is dwelling on it or analysing with the rehab experts. Mood swings still excessive. Feeling of weakness in the legs not happening so much. Cannot lift much weight still – 3–4 kgs is the limit.*

Cooking continued to be a good distraction, but now I felt it was time to plan travel again. After my scan in June, I was reassured that flying would do me no harm. My brain, I was told, had puffed out to its normal size and there had been no more bleeding. So, after postponing our air tickets for months, we finally said we would go to Australia to see family and friends. The dates were set: June the 28th to July the 13th, four months since my fall and three months since the second operation.

In the meantime, Kate, who dealt with the computer, mail, errands and some of the many chores for two or three days a week at Mark's office, and who had been keeping an eye on my company too, had to leave. What would I do? The big issue was always getting help that both Mark and I felt comfortable with.

22 JUNE. *What an interminable nightmare. It has been downhill for the past two weeks, culminating in this living hell of strange sensations. Then Ishy — almond biscuits decorated by the wooden rose biscuit printer — order and routine, protection from the family and friends, soothing.*

Ishy was a traveller from the Isle of Muck in Scotland — a tiny island inhabited by only ten families. She had come to New Zealand to heal after sadness in her family, and because she was looking for a theatre experience she sought me out in Christchurch. Someone I had taught as an adult student rang to ask me if I could work with Ishy and give her some help in finding a place in the theatre industry. After I had explained my circumstances, he asked me, 'Please see her at least. She's a very nice young woman.' And so Ishy came into my life one winter afternoon, looking for a new direction, and found me utterly lost and in a black hole.

She arrived at what was a desperately low time for me. Bella, our large black canine friend, had disappeared one dark, stormy afternoon after going outside for a walk. She wasn't discovered for six weeks. When he saw her body the vet believed that she had died instantly, hit by a car on the road above our home. To add to this, it was midwinter, Mark's and my relationship was straining at the seams, and I was exhausted.

Ishy had energy, warmth and sympathy. She was quiet, yet incredibly practical and able. Miraculously, she did dishes and prepared food in our open-plan house without hurting my sensitised brain. She was sensible and strong, but gentle and quiet. She managed to slide in between all the jarring family relationships and just be there for me. Ishy saw me through another phase of healing.

Her driving was the scariest thing. I tried to be a passenger a few times but this was the least therapeutic part of our relationship. Ishy was, as she put it, dyslexic with directions and signage of all kinds, and driving – which she had only just mastered in her late twenties – was not an activity either she or her passengers could be comfortable with.

Ishy gave me two to three intense months of support, both in the house and with the accounts and my business, before the spring lambs in the high country called and the boyfriend arrived. She wanted to work on a farm and help with the lambing, so she moved on, leaving behind wonderful memories.

At this stage I was still very uncomfortable in a car, let alone an aircraft. My tolerance for speed was very limited and I found acceleration from stationary especially uncomfortable. How was it going to be travelling down a runway, then rising quickly to a very high altitude? Mark thought that a practise was an idea with merit. He drove me into the country and tried to simulate an aircraft take-off with the car – not good.

Armed with medical confirmation that I was safe to travel, a huge will to get back to the patterns of my previous life, and an even bigger desire to be near my daughter and grandchildren, I prepared for our departure to Australia.

In my past life, packing was a very insignificant event. I was efficient and fast, and would think nothing of throwing a bag together the day or even the night before I travelled. Now, I had to have new strategies. Time was essential and I had plenty of that. I took pleasure in sorting and choosing the summer clothes I would take to Australia, laying them out. It took such a long time to pack my bag for that first post-operation journey – perhaps ten days or so.

Finally the day came. I can remember little about the journey now. What I do recall is the pain and pressure in my head as we lifted off. I had taken Panadol, Mark was holding me, and my hands were pressed to my temples to block out the vibrations and noise. Tears were pouring down my face. We had been upgraded to business class, so I had physical comfort, and when we settled at cruising altitude the pressure and pain abated. I collapsed back into my seat, exhausted emotionally but fine. I had done it. When I had rested for a few minutes, the sense of achievement kicked in. I was so happy, the trapped feeling gone for a few hours. Mark and I were on our way for a break. I was going to get better.

Sydney airport seemed familiar yet different: it was as though things had been shifted or rearranged very subtly. Patterns were still a nightmare for me. Those who designed carpets for airports and other large public places certainly never had brain-injured people in mind.

Sydney, that first time in my new life, meant delight – at being in a hotel, at having no demands placed on me. My memories are of relaxation, luxury, cotton-wool protection, the Botanic Gardens, the warmth of the sun. I could walk with assistance from Mark but then needed to rest on seats in the gardens, which brought tears, and yet more tears, of frustration. But when Mark left me alone for fifteen to thirty minutes, sitting at a café across from the hotel with a blanket over my legs to ward off the chill in the winter air, I was fascinated by the light reflected on the warm sandstone buildings, which contrasted so beautifully with the sharp modern glass constructions alongside them. I was elated and excited by such heightened visual perceptions – when I could control the input. I was panicked and emotionally upset by stimulus that was beyond my control. I needed to cut down the input, and would have to learn new strategies to do so.

When a friend suggested that we go to an afternoon dance performance at one of the Opera House theatres, I rashly booked. It was expensive, but I saw it as another first in my rehabilitation process. I'd been a theatre person for thirty years: I wanted to test myself in this environment again.

This first theatre experience only five months into my recovery process wasn't a positive one. My recovering brain didn't like the vibrations of the didgeridoo. My reaction was embarrassing: tears pouring down my cheeks, hands held up to my face, fingers outspread so I could peer through them and obtain a limited view of the stage. There was only one performer I could watch. I had enjoyed theatre for so much of my life, relishing in the passion, the conjunction of the visual and aural. The extreme sensory receptivity, once a joy to me, was now a nightmare. But I could see that continuing to expose myself to doses of complexity was definitely the way to go, so despite my distress we went back to the show after half-time. My tolerance was still low and I couldn't say I enjoyed it, but I got through it. There was, and there continues to be, a feeling of exhilaration – 'I did it!' – after each new achievement.

I understood my aural problems better when I received an audiologist's report in April the following year. The test results showed 'reduced loudness tolerance in the right ear in particular' and that I had 'some difficulties with processing auditory information'. My problems with hyperacusis (hyper-hearing) were causing me 'to avoid many situations and withdraw from various aspects of her life'.

At first, my achievements had been major things, like walking without a walking frame (after four days) and lying on my right side for the first time (at three months). Then it had been walking the 300 metres to the beach and back, or getting through a whole twenty-four hours without my eye jamming shut (after eight months). There had also been my first outing in the car and my first visit to the supermarket with a helper.

Now, three months after my second operation, I was en route from Sydney to friends in Noosa, via Maroochydore. This flight wasn't as alarming as the first one from New Zealand to Sydney

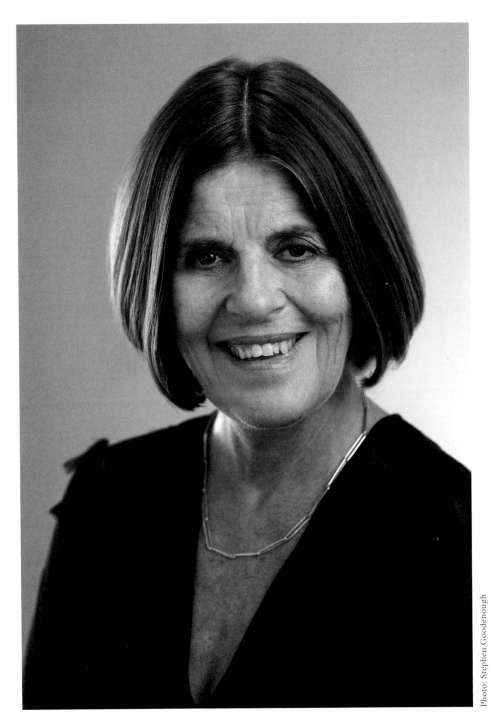

Grateful to be alive, February 2008

Photo: Stephen Goodenough

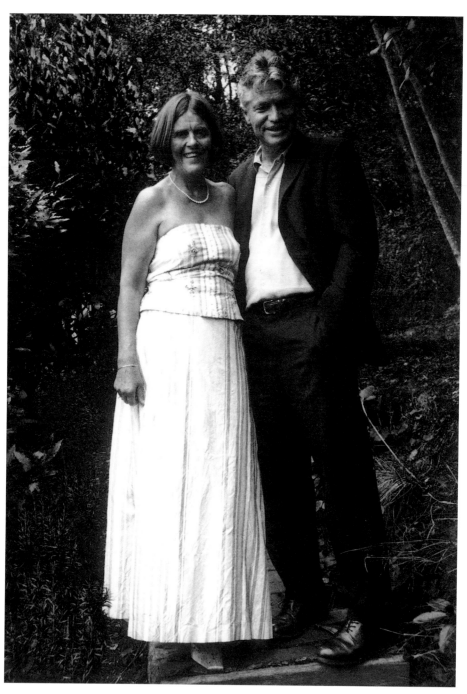

With Mark on our way to the wedding celebration, 7 February 2004

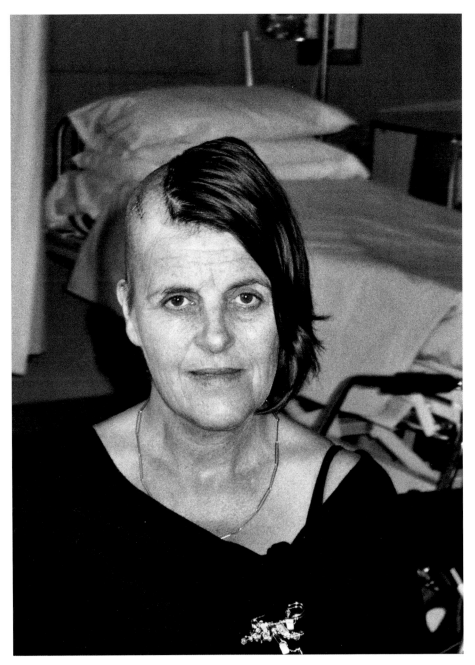

A week after the second surgical procedure, Christchurch Public Hospital, April 2004

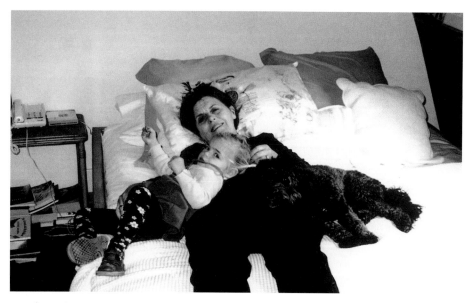

Resting at home with granddaughter Lili and Lui the dog, 2005

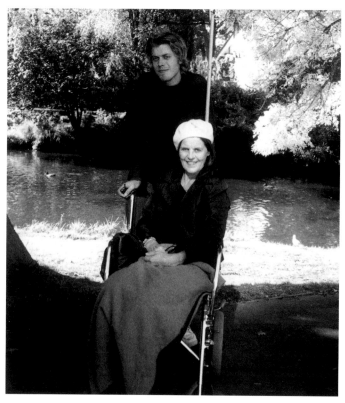

Escape from the ward: an outing around the park with son, Ollie, April 2004

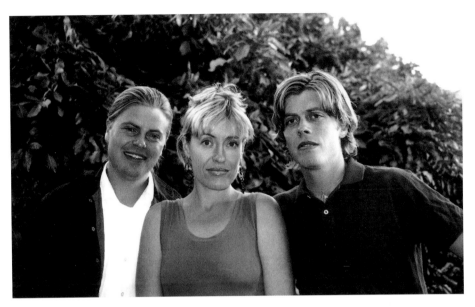

Our children (left to right) Mischa, Aimee and Ollie, 2005

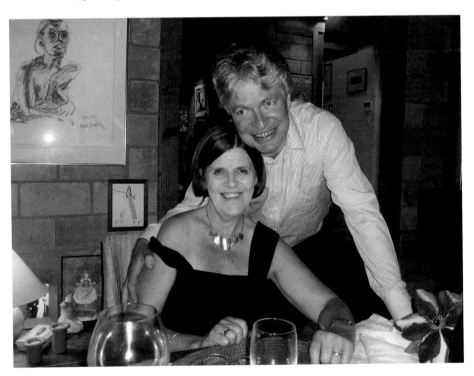

At home 'Ribbonwood', Governors Bay, November 2007

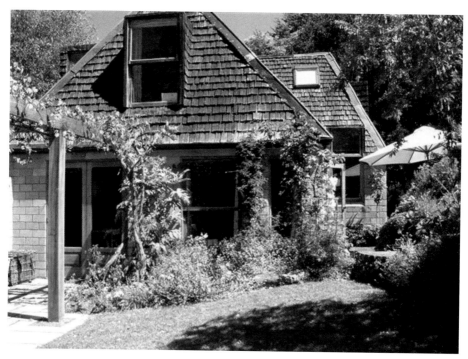

'Ribbonwood', Governors Bay

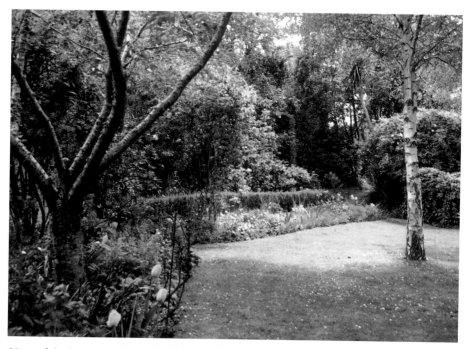

View of the bottom garden at 'Ribbonwood', Governors Bay

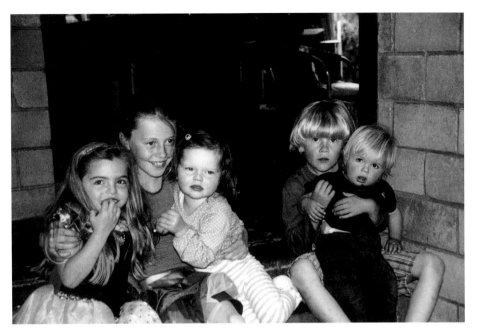

Grandchildren (left to right) Lili, Sophia, Grace, Arlo and Iñaki, December 2007

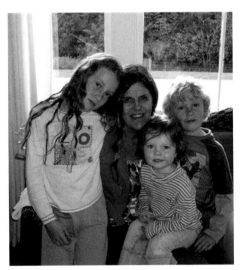

In Cambridge with grandchildren (left to right) Sophia, Grace and Arlo, 2007

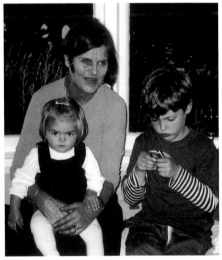

With grandchildren Lili (on knee) and Reuben, May 2004

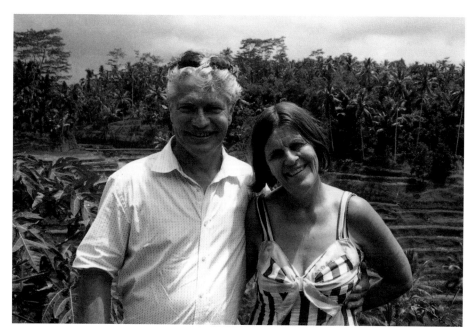

In Bali with Mark, December 2007

had been. I knew the routine now: have plenty to eat and drink before departure; wear sunglasses in the airport to cut down on sensory overload; stick with the bag trolley as long as possible so you can lean on it, looking nonchalant; sit near a window on the flight so you can put pillows around you and sleep; and swallow a couple of Panadol before take-off.

It was wonderful to be in the warmth of a Queensland winter and the home of a loving friend. It was strange to be revisiting places and people I knew so well, yet that seemed so different, often in subtle ways. Walking, always such a joy, was now so limited. I would stop mid-journey and have to sit down, often crying, then be brought back by car. My friends Alan and Alison were so compassionate and caring, and such fun. Evening mealtimes were always a delight, but only as long as I had had adequate rest during the afternoon to enjoy the good food, a glass of wine and the great conversation. I tired quickly, but I was part of things again. I had always loved fine food, and my appetite for perfection and beauty in all things was fed in this environment, surrounded by Alan's artworks inside and the grand eucalypts outside. And my body began to tan, though my face still had a strange pallor.

Then it was on to Townsville in north Queensland, to my dearest daughter Aimee, her husband HJ and the grandchildren. I experienced another set of shocks as I realised how little tolerance I now had for the noise and clamour of family life.

We had booked to stay near the family so we could have frequent access to them, but not be overwhelmed by them – or them by me. This worked extremely well. I could maintain a daily schedule of exercise and rest while enjoying the delights of grandparenting my darling Arlo and Sophia again, and the companionship of my daughter.

But the happy times with the children could cause me to deteriorate rapidly, like a child who's had a busy day and gets beside itself. I would go white, feel faint and then tears would pour forth uncontrollably. Of course, my poor grandchildren were upset to see me like this. Even many months later, when I went back for a second visit, Sophia was heard to say, 'Is this the old Granny coming back? Because I don't like the new Granny. I want my old Granny back.' I wanted her back too. I wanted to be able to enjoy these small people, to pick them up in my arms and cuddle them, to run on the beach with them.

It was at this stage that I started to have my running dreams. I would be convinced that I could run again, only to be confronted by the painful reality when I woke up and headed out that I couldn't run, and that I was still challenged by walking.

So it was in the warmth of Townsville in July that a new phase of my recovery began – swimming, walking (for perhaps fifteen minutes in the morning with Mark supporting me) and starting to read novels again. While I was there I developed strategies that helped me to rejoin some of my previous life. If I became upset I would go immediately to a quiet room on my own, take Panadol and lie flat on a bed. If an eye mask was available I would use it, or if not I would just put a towel or a cloth over my eyes, to shut out all external stimuli as much as possible. I would cry, then rest. This procedure usually had quick results.

All the lying about and frequent eating was playing havoc with my formerly trim body, but I knew that the most important thing at this stage was to relax my brain and to feel good and not stressed. If eating tasty food helped to deliver this result then I would continue the regime. In addition, I made a pact with myself that I would continue walking a little each day.

Townsville was a wonderful success. I felt a real sense of achievement as we flew out towards Sydney on our way back to New Zealand.

Twenty-one

1 AUGUST. *I'm starting to climb out of the hole. The trip to Oz was a brilliant pick-me-up. I can't believe how long this recovery is taking. I still can't lift over 4 kg but I'm walking further with the aid of a walking stick and am more confident on my own. Visual disturbance is still present, though. I can't tolerate confusing or moving patterns, blue lights or flashing lights of any colour. Loud noise can make me feel sick and very mentally disturbed. I'm still taking Panadol to calm me down most days.*

14 AUGUST. *It's Saturday, and I'm in Little Pigeon Bay with Ishy and Lui, my new little dog. The waves are crashing into the stones. The high tide is on the return now, the sun not yet up. It's good to be here but also a reminder that I'm not yet the old me. I still experience the symptoms of vertigo, and overstimulation causes extreme discomfort and panic. I must have a boring routine or else! I joked with Ishy yesterday that the surgeon has caused a short circuit in the rewiring, resulting in my not being able to indulge in the passions of my previous life, i.e. animated discussion, analysis, anger, excitement, laughter. Anything with too much feeling seems to be a circuit-breaker and I'm stopped in my tracks. I can do only one thing at a time. The surgeon, joking, had said, 'You're now like a man.'*

My walking was improving, however. The circuit-breaker was taking longer to kick in. Early mornings were the best for energy, particularly for telephone conversations. I noticed how much I was using television or film to dull myself. In Pigeon Bay there was no music, no TV. Magazines worked better to calm me than novels. My God, enforced dumbing down – how horrific.

Conflict was unbearable: my head reacted, pressure built up and I had to walk away. Ishy thought I should walk away from all my responsibilities for a while and go somewhere warm where I could just concentrate on getting well. It was nice in theory, but how would I cope without my caregivers, and without my combative companion and lover? I would miss Mark's presence hugely, though not his preoccupation with his business. Sometimes I thought that perhaps I was just expecting too much, and I probably was, being so absorbed in my own needs.

15 AUGUST. *What do I need to achieve?*
- *To have confidence and trust in myself again, both physically and mentally.*
- *To get to know my body again and tone it and get it functioning safely so it won't let me down.*
- *To be happy to be alone, and to feel safe.*
- *To become unconscious again of what's going on inside my head.*

As a result of conversations with my therapists and other medical staff, I was programmed to think I would be better by August or September. I remember saying to myself, Well, that will be the end of ACC assistance. It's been so nice of them to help me, but I'll be back at work by then. My office door in town had been closed for months – now would be the time to open it to new beginnings.

My work with the students at Christchurch Medical School was scheduled to begin in mid-August and to run for twelve two-hour sessions. I was nervous, but also excited about going back into the real world. Soon I would be driving, soon I would be teaching, soon I would be casting again. I would once more be managing the myriad things for Mark's work. There had been a blip of about six months, but hey, I could have been overseas.

Now, looking back, I think I was right — at least about being able to reinstate my business. I could have kick-started it all again if I'd been able to get back to work properly in August 2004 after a six-month break. But it wasn't to be.

5 SEPTEMBER. *Achievements at six months:*

- *Can tolerate more weight-carrying capacity, probably up to about 5 kg now.*
- *Can tolerate car travel — fewer symptoms. Still fear of cars coming too close. Big frights.*
- *Can tolerate telephone conversations — more frequent and for longer.*
- *Independence increasing, e.g. can go into café now and order.*
- *Can go into public bathrooms and feel okay; can be dropped off, e.g. outside hospital and can walk to class (tonight the first time from the kerbside). Still feel like I'm going to fall over and feel sick, but get there.*
- *Can go to the pictures and watch more without feeling too dizzy — less time shutting my eyes. Still need to limit vision and sound with earplugs and hands shielding eyes, and sit in the back row so I can lean on the wall.*
- *Can walk on my own to the beach and beyond with Lui on lead. Exhausted on return but achieve it. Have done it for the first time with no one in the house waiting for me.*
- *Drove car out of drive and to wharf and back. Had huge difficulties reversing but essentially achieved the basic mechanics. Didn't have to deal with any traffic at all, though!*
- *Have flown unaccompanied from Auckland to Christchurch. Escorted to plane and off plane.*

These were all big steps forward compared with what I could manage two months before.

14 SEPTEMBER. *I'm in a house at Wakefield Quay in Nelson. I flew here unaccompanied and, another first, I'm settled in on my own. I wanted to achieve this but I'm not feeling comfortable in myself.*

15 SEPTEMBER. *An old school friend said to me yesterday, 'Well Rosie, I can't imagine you of all people, always on the go, stopped in your tracks.' But then she added, 'At least with your life so full and rich with experiences, you've got a lot to think about as you wait to get better.'*

That is so true. I do have so much to think back on. Of course, I didn't think of my present situation as an end to my old life, but simply as rather a long blip – time to reflect, time to dream and plan, time to learn new skills, time to listen.

The flax leaves outside my window in Nelson moved in the breeze. The sunlight made patterns on my floor. My mother's comment that morning by phone came back to me: 'You're taking time to collect yourself before moving on again.' And I looked at what I still had. My senses weren't dulled; rather they were heightened. I relished the exquisite tastes of fine food, lovingly grown and prepared. I revelled in my keen sense of smell – pungent flowering currants, spring violets, jasmine, daphne, and cosmetic delights such as lavender to gentle my spirit and verbena to awaken me. The salty sea smells comforted me, as did Lui, with his curly little dog body, and the warm smell on my husband's neck – sometimes a whiff of almond or lavender shaving cream, sometimes just him.

My hearing was now so acute that it could discomfort me, but it could also delight: the pure, clear notes of the bellbird and the tui – such clarity – and the perfection of some of the classical pieces in my music collection. Hearing was the last sense I learned to cope with after the operation, and it took months before I could listen to music. Even now I can only rarely immerse myself in the listening experience as I used to, and only in controlled situations, preferably when I'm alone without any other stimuli distracting me.

I remembered working at the Drama Centre in its heyday, when the office computer was at the edge of its ability to store more information and printers were belching forth script. Happy sounds of excited learning coming from the students, and from the props room came the sounds of building and creating – the magic of theatre. The round table in my office was the site of so many animated conversations. Here, hours and months were spent putting together the dreams and putting down the facts to bring the funding in. The joy of that room for me – my life for up to eight or nine hours a day, often seven days a week – was the discipline and the independence it offered.

This was my life away from the other me, the wife, mother, grandmother and home-maker, yet the two were interwoven – merging, seemingly effortless, effortlessly seamless. Like an athlete building up strength and stamina for the Olympics, I had built up my capabilities, my capacity to cope with the long days and the demands made on me. My stamina had been incredible in those complex, variety-filled days.

I used to tackle finance in the first part of the day when the house was quiet and the phones did not demand my attention. Next came the writing and creation of ideas, then my midday dash from Governors Bay into the city offices to deal with the administrative tasks and join the busy team. I would respond to telephone calls and electronic and paper mail, and somewhere in all of this would prepare for my classes – my greatest love and the greatest drain on my energy. I seldom had more than half an hour off throughout my long days. The teaching load would vary, but typically I would spend five hours in front of classes in the late afternoon and early evening. Then there was the extra teaching –

daytime teaching in schools, plus tertiary teacher training – and the businesses I worked with and their staff training.

Not only that, but casting work also came and went, bringing intense, short periods of chaos and frenetic activity. These castings fed the dreams of so many students and their families – to be seen on television or to be in a movie. We worked hard on some of those movies. I could see clearly in my mind's eye 250-plus schoolgirls crushing stairwells and hallways, as four or five hairdressers worked at top speed, shearing their locks as they lined up, uncomplaining for hours, excited to be extras in Peter Jackson's *Heavenly Creatures*.

Now, I felt exhausted and bewildered merely thinking of it all. As I said to Mark, 'It's incredible what I did each day, but I expected to be looking back on it at seventy-five, not fifty-five. I've still got so much to do.'

Twenty-two

Work had been an integral part of my life – not just something I did from nine to five, but the activity that gave me a daily framework and purpose. I loved (mostly) what I did, so when there was an abrupt halt as a result of the surgeries, I realised that work, in its usual format, wasn't possible. I continued, however, to try to deal with the paperwork that arrived on my bed. The figures on the cash flows somehow gave me a feeling of purpose and control, and to my relief I found I could still enjoy numbers.

During my first year of recovery I wasn't able to measure my work abilities. I was trying to run before I could walk, trying to manage high-level executive functioning before I could cope with getting through a day at home in an undiminished, unfatigued way.

To their credit, my ACC manager at the time and my therapists allowed me to try to explore my old work roles. This let me discover my limitations and make my own decisions about letting aspects of my work world go, rather than them telling me I wouldn't be able to cope. I remain grateful for this approach.

I made many attempts to go back to what had been my major occupation before the injury: doing the financial planning and strategy work for my husband's business. This work was always intense, and after the surgery the pressure became unbearable.

I did realise that a trip to Vancouver for an event to do with my arts work some six weeks after the second operation wasn't possible.

I couldn't, however, accept that I was losing the other part of that business – casting. Casting jobs came in as they always had – by email or telephone. I never met the people behind these communications, so why or how would they know I was any different?

I remember a call coming in on the mobile – 'Hi, I'm calling from Tokyo. Can you do an urgent casting for us?' I went onto automatic pilot, felt the adrenalin of the job kicking in and responded without thinking: when, where, who, how many, time line, etc. I functioned pretty well for this five-minute telephone conversation. I was accustomed to being asked for the impossible: finding people who in those minutes on the phone you couldn't visualise finding, filming them today or tomorrow, and then having the finished product couriered or emailed away by 6 PM the next day. As a casting director you kept your cool exterior, you committed to the job, you got on with it and you supplied the product on time, making it – the casting tape or email attachments – as accurate as possible.

Approximately half an hour after I had committed to doing this job, I suddenly realised the huge gap between my desire to be back doing what I knew and loved, and my new state of being – the new me who couldn't take too much excitement, who needed quiet and rests, whose legs became like lead and whose system threatened to shut down. It was ridiculous to consider doing the job. With great sadness I picked up the phone, rang the contact number and told the person, 'I'm sorry, I shouldn't have committed to this job. I'm recovering from brain surgery and I'm not up to doing this work again yet.' The usual questions, of course, came from the stranger on the line: 'Oh my God, you poor thing, how terrible. So who can do the job for us?'

After twelve months or so I did try another casting job. There was a little more run-in time – time to organise a crew of helpers, advise my therapists, train an assistant. The job was top-heavy on helpers, but never mind, I was back in the driver's seat. The project was an ad pushing for more custom at a local family eatery. The script struck me as being particularly lacking in honesty and integrity, but so what, I was working again; I had a framework again – briefly.

There were children to cast, and smiling mums and dads and grandparents who all loved and wanted to go and eat at the restaurant. I made strategies to cope with the pressures of the build up to casting day and the event itself. Premises were hired with an extra space at the back so I could withdraw and lie down when necessary. The calls (times for auditions) were made slightly further apart and the number of children per call were limited. We tried to keep the atmosphere in the audition space calm, quiet and organised in between takes.

At first I was happy. There were a few moments when I forgot what had happened to me – I'm on my way, I thought. This is what I need, a reminder of my old life. I can do it. So what if I require so many support crew that economically it can't work? Fundamentally what matters is that I feel successful and I'm contributing.

It was perhaps an hour into the initial day that I first felt the pressure. My confidence began to wane. I started to lose patience rapidly with each group of children coming through – not the way to get a good performance out of them for those seconds needed on camera so that the ad director would be able to make an informed choice about final casting. I was exhausted, over-whelmed and anxious about the product, and had to go in and out of the room in order to rest and withdraw from the noise. I was unable to ensure the quality or the evenness of the auditions. I recall snapping at one of the mothers when her child just wouldn't cooperate. I retreated again. It was a very strange day. We got the tape away on the scheduled flight and the company seemed satisfied, but the product was the result of the contributions of many people; in my eyes, I hadn't coped with my role as a casting director. I haven't tried again since.

The new role I had been offered by the Christchurch Medical School before the accident – teaching fifth-year medical students communication skills – was another exciting work project. Seven months after the surgeries, intellectually I was willing to give the teaching a go, but would my condition allow me to survive the classroom situation for a two-hour stretch? Before the classes started I was asked to attend a talk in the lecture theatre and sit in front of the students with the other tutors.

It was such a bizarre feeling, sitting there and looking up at the sea of faces. I was required to speak briefly about what I was offering – it had to be interesting in order to tempt these busy students to want to add this rather nebulous subject of drama to their already overloaded week.

Here I was promising something, but could I deliver? Should I tell them now what had happened? Was it fraudulent not to, or was I making too much of my condition if I did tell them?

I managed two two-hour sessions a week in a three-week block, then some more sessions interspersed with breaks over a total period of about ten to twelve weeks – just twelve classes in all. This was regarded as a work trial. So what happened? First, whatever my emotional state, I got there each time. Sometimes I was a bit late, underestimating how long it would take to make it from the car to the lift to the teaching room. I was escorted to the room for the first few sessions, then managed by myself. I was very happy to be in a teaching environment again.

Student numbers per class never exceeded thirteen, which felt like enough anyway. I made a decision to reveal to each of the six groups during their first session with me that I was recovering from a surgical procedure and suffering some vestibular disturbance. I kept the issue as light as I could, while at the same time making quite clear to them what my physical limitations were.

The vestibular system regulates automatic eye movements,

body position and balance; when it's malfunctioning, as can easily happen with a brain injury, the result is vertigo and disequilibrium. The damage can be peripheral or central. The peripheral sensory receptors detect motion, whereas central damage affects structures such as the brain stem, cerebellum and cortex, which are involved in the integration and perception of balance, determining exactly where the movements around us occur. Sufferers have difficulty in coping with a high intensity of visual or auditory stimuli – such as noise, people, movement and traffic – and 'sensory overload' occurs. People with central vestibular damage recover much more slowly and may never fully return to normal.

I felt like I was in a strange dream. Some weeks I was elated by the pleasure of being in front of students again: there was a sense of achievement and pleasure at interacting with bright young people. Other days I was left with feelings of self-doubt and self-consciousness. I would withdraw and flail around with self-pity, grief and a feeling of loss; it seemed impossible to picture a work-world future.

It was during the second year of my rehabilitation that I attempted to return to the other training job I'd done for many years – teaching in fifty-hour blocks for the Christchurch College of Education. I was responsible for three papers for drama studies teachers who were upgrading to a degree or adding to their professional development.

The course had been re-advertised without my knowledge, and suddenly I was rung and told I had students – could I work with them? My initial reaction was, Great, I'm still wanted. Then, as usual, reality struck and I realised that it was impossible for me to fulfil the requirements. Many compromises were made by assisting staff and by the students, and I agreed to lecture and direct a drastically shortened course. I employed two people to assist and shadow me, who could take over where necessary. This required extra work on my part, explaining to them what needed to be done, and it added to the stress at times, since the course became inconsistent as it was continually affected by staff changes.

The group of students was small, numbering ten to twelve. It was so good arriving that first day, dressed for work and going into an environment I had known well, but strange not be to be able to walk unaided to the room.

Things went well at first – for perhaps an hour – and then I needed to rest. I made a rest area for myself in the room. Most of the students were okay with this, though at least one felt some-what short-changed by having a teacher giving instruction from a prone position. It must have seemed very odd.

There was a lot of pressure on everyone. The course require-ments were eventually fulfilled, but the cost to relationships with colleagues supporting me, to my family and to my ongoing need to improve the fatigue symptoms were too high to warrant repeating this situation. This was very distressing for me to adjust to, because intellectually I loved being back in front of students. I was so excited by reactivating areas of my teaching expertise, so happy to be facilitating learning in others again. But it wasn't really workable, emotionally, physically or economically. I'm grateful to all those who helped me trial this work.

Being a troubleshooter was a challenge I had always thrived on, but now any trouble, any conflict, any pressure, had dire personal effects. There were constant attempts in that first year after sur-gery to connect again with Mark's business. I would have times of energy and then, like a skittle, just fall over.

The trial back in Mark's office took place during the latter part of year one and continued for part of year two. I went twice a week for three hours. The problems that occurred then are much the same now. I have to put strategies in place: a good rest before I go to the office, a careful driver on the way in, snacks and a hot drink on arrival, a calm and organised approach to whatever needs to be done, being seated near a wall so I can lean against it when tired, sitting so that I can see everyone else without having to turn from left to right too often, and keeping turned away from strong light or light coming through slim-line Venetian blinds. Provided all environmental factors are as controlled as possible, I will survive two hours, but the minute intensity increases during a discussion, or if conflict occurs, I fall apart. I'm no longer resilient or reliable.

I feel able to take in complex discussions to a point, then I cease to receive the information adequately and require a lot of explanation. This slows everything down, to the frustration of the other participants, I'm sure. I'm exhilarated, as always, by rigorous intellectual discussion, but I simply can't maintain the pace and have to rest at home for many hours afterwards. I feel distressed, disoriented and fearful about my future.

Twenty-three

19 SEPTEMBER. *Today I went back to Accident and Emergency, feeling as though I was fading with pain and exhaustion and disorientation. They scanned me again. They were delightful to me. I'm still teaching the med students – only a few classes to go now. It scares me before I get there but being with the students actually focuses me and makes me remember another time. But my confidence wavers, my moods are very on edge, my tolerances are low. For the first time I feel angry about what has happened.*

23 SEPTEMBER. *What a rollercoaster it has been over recent days and weeks. That disgusting feeling of why am I not better yet, why can't I be the old me. The tears, the rages, the feeling of not being able to make it. I had to stop the swimming after only two visits to the pool. I got pins and needles badly. I went to the osteopath and it helped a bit. I find that when I break my mundane routines it freaks me out and I'm distressed for hours, sometimes days.*

4 OCTOBER. *Mark struggled to keep his cool with me today. My emotions were raw – they're much improved eight months down the track but today I was up and down and all over the place. I felt so trapped and vulnerable and my 'nut', as my friend Alison described it, drove me crazy with discomfort: immovable, it had a mind of its own.*

At fifty-five I was humbled, dependent and completely reliant on a husband who struggled with being so needed, a husband whose business worries continued to preoccupy him –

who worked from home, long and odd hours on the computer and telephone, tapping late into the night in an office too close to my bedroom and talking loudly at all hours to people in other time zones. There was humiliation, anger and frustration on both sides. We struggled to keep the memories alive of how we were before the bang on the head. Each day we tried to make a new life.

After my afternoon sleep or rest and the invention of the evening meal, I would try to work a little – maybe on my writing. My eyesight was still very variable – sometimes the vision was clear, sometimes not. I would go very pale and need to sit or stop.

5 OCTOBER. *I'm in New Caledonia (the trip has been rescheduled from July). The warmth and the peace are thawing me – problems are dissipating. Today I want to resume my writing. I feel so improved that I have the courage to look back again. It is 6.30 AM. The sun appeared half an hour ago. Bird life announced the day – doves cooing in the background. I contemplate the changes that have occurred to me and the shift in my perceptions.*

The outcome of this bang on the head wasn't all bad when I considered the benefits I'd received. Always one for observing, I now had time to do so as never before. I had run my life at full speed, not allowing any gaps for contemplation. If there was a gap, I would fill it. Sundays, for example, had always seemed like gaps – yawning chasms where family should have been. If they weren't with me, which was most of the time since they lived in different geographical locations, I would invite people in – lots of people. It was fun and stimulating, but also exhausting.

The second a project I was on began to conclude, I would create a new one. Always stretching the limits, I seemed to be obsessed with cramming my life full, always aware of the short time we all have in this world. I didn't regret these experiences – quite the opposite. Without that life behind me I would not have been so accepting of, excited by and grateful for aspects of the new one. If I hadn't experienced things full on, how could I ever have appreciated slowing down?

14 NOVEMBER. *This morning I turned the Raoul Dufy calendar to November (two weeks into the month, a bit late). Here was this figure stepping out from a French artist's palette – big movement forward. It's me, I thought. This is November, forward I go. October was love and tenderness and intimacy, New Caledonia. Early November was another trip to Sydney and Townsville, friendship and family, love and warmth. Now November – independence, strength, moving forward into somewhere new.*

2 DECEMBER. *Since the operation I have little or no tolerance for some behaviour. If there were nuances of discomfort or recurring suggestions of a friendship or relationship not being quite right before the fall, these aspects become magnified for me after the accident.*

This change in me led to sharp endings of some old friendships. I felt that if someone really cared about me, they would continue to care after such an alteration in my circumstances – a bit like the old 'in sickness and in health' vow. Unless the people around me could acknowledge this, and accept that I was now different, I couldn't move on into the future with them. I suppose I set the standards very high, and when my expectations were not met, I froze and put up a wall.

Other things placed a strain on old friendships, such as my reaction to being driven. I was – and still am – so sensitive to being bumped about in a car or accelerating too fast from stationary. When this happened I felt personally and irrationally hurt, as if the other person wasn't caring for me and was instead ignoring my need for gentleness. And I grew so tired of having to explain such reactions. They were all so subtle and internal that unless I turned pale or looked as though I was about to fall over, I believed my family and friends thought I was playing on my condition.

Twenty-four

I was so excited as the day approached for my driving assessment, in December 2004. After all, it was eight months since my last surgery and my friend Maxine, who I met during my first stay in hospital, had been driving since six months after her operation. My car, which had been sitting idle in the garage, was cleaned and Mark came home from work to drive me to Burwood, where the testing would take place.

In November I had gone to Burwood to take the off-road assessment and had passed these tests. For the on-road assessment I had two assessors in the car with me. Unfortunately, I experienced significant fatigue and head pain as the assessment progressed, and this impaired my performance. I drove too slowly and I didn't look around me enough. So although I was judged as having a 'calm measured approach to driving' and 'excellent physical control of the vehicle', it was deemed inappropriate for me to return to driving at this stage. I was so exhausted after just twenty minutes of the forty-five-minute assessment that I didn't actually care about the conclusion. I knew I wasn't ready.

As I write this it is late 2006 and I'm still not driving. This is difficult to accept. It seems a strange system that allows people who have had brain surgery for a cerebral haemorrhage or tumour to be back at the wheel six months later, yet those whose condition was the result of an accident must undergo assessment and achieve particular goals before getting back in the driving seat.

I have attempted to drive again since that test back in 2004. Twice, in times of immense frustration, I've got into my car early on a Sunday morning when there is little or no traffic on the road, and headed off up the hill to the Summit Road. What exhilaration it was to be behind the wheel, my own boss, and to gaze down at beautiful Lyttelton Harbour. The joy the first time was huge. The big problem was that when I had to get out of the car after this drive of perhaps ten minutes' duration, I couldn't walk. All my energy had gone into the concentrated effort of driving.

It was another year before I tried to repeat this adventure. This time I went prepared with a thermos of tea, food snacks, my dog Lui for moral support and plenty of warm clothes. And I was successful. I enjoyed a short walk, then a rest, then the descent home. I did find it tricky though, as other cars had started to use the road by the time I set off on my return.

Burwood requires me to achieve certain results before they will test me again. An ophthalmologist's report must indicate a set level of ability with visual plotting and tracking, and the neuropsychologist must report on progress made with multi-tasking, visual processing and fatigue. Of these, fatigue is the 'biggie'.

I did see the ophthalmologist, finally, one year later, and also the neuropsychologist. Unfortunately, the ophthalmology report revealed problems with ocular movement. I lacked the ability to move my eyes quickly, owing to 'damage to the parietal region and areas of higher visual function and particularly visual/body space on top of the vestibular damage'.

I hope I will drive again. I look forward to that independence. My son now has my car.

Twenty-five

It was January the 25th, 2005 and I was back in idyllic Little Pigeon Bay, staying in a bach there. The day before I had been for a walk with my companion and friend Jani. We had gone along the gravel road for a few hundred metres, and then onto the grassy peninsula that sloped gently out into the ocean. I was excited to be walking and in one of my favourite places. Then I had a memory of being there about six months ago on my last visit. I had achieved this before, I was sure of it, so why wasn't I independent now? Why wasn't I walking without a stick? Why wasn't I running?

The return from the peninsula walk was slow. I needed a lot of support and I felt absolutely drained, and sad, about the loss of the old me, about the waiting. Obviously these thoughts had affected me deeply, because the previous night I had dreamed that I was walking just fine and driving again, fast and confident, and moving my head with ease.

Patience and hope: two old-fashioned words often given as names for children to wear their whole life, but still descriptive of a state of being – perseverance, endurance, expectation. When you're recovering from brain injury the experts all tell you that it will be a long process. Yes it is, and patience is required in large doses, from you the sufferer, and from the family and friends around you. Another ingredient must be thrown in – hope, which creeps back in because you feel okay for a while, satisfied, content. And hope combats the dismay as you find yourself sliding backwards on some days. What other illness or injury would have you move forward one month, only to stay still for another two or three months, and then go right back to where you were six months before?

If you break your leg there's a progression forward. You're temporarily disabled as the leg begins to heal. Then the plaster comes off and you deal with the weak leg. Slowly, with exercise and discipline, you build your leg back into condition, depending on the severity of the break. It may not be quite the same as it was before, but nevertheless you walk again, you run again. But with a brain injury, that's not what happens.

I found various occupations that worked as therapy for me. They included fixing things – those special items that had got broken over the years and then been tucked away for mending one day. So out they came. First, three wooden African birds, chewed by Bella in her puppy phase. I filled the chewed marks with wood filler, then sanded and painted. It was entirely satisfying to see the regeneration of these loved treasures bought with my son long ago from a shop in Paris. I managed numerous fix-its, including some ceramic birds, which needed a lot of work. I even did some stitching, on a doll that was bleeding wood shavings after another dog-chewing accident. Somehow this focusing on, and re-creation of, something known proved most therapeutic, and I was surprised to find that I had previously untapped talents. Fixing the items also gave me time to muse on their origins and to recall the adventures that accompanied their purchase.

At this time I was also writing as much as I could. The process, while satisfying, was exhausting to my brain. I couldn't use the computer, so handwriting in notebooks became the method. My typist, Jeanette, was truly amazing at deciphering my entries, which were never in a neat progression, but jumped from place to place and from notebook to notebook – the brown one, the pink one, the gold-covered one with white feathers glued on, given to me by my healer friend Eva. The process continued – back would come the typing, both in hard copy and by email.

I then began to collate the bits. During the first eighteen months this was the most difficult process, getting things into order in terms of tense and chronology. Before my injury, this was an exercise I was extremely good at, but now I would start with the best of intentions and end up feeling confused, beaten and unable to continue. When I look now at the reports from the speech–language therapist, I see the deficits that were measured probably also caused impairment in this area of organisational skill. I do believe that with constant practice this skill has improved, although when I'm tired it can still turn to custard.

Cooking continued to be useful in calming my troubled brain, and was not too demanding physically, especially as my galley-style kitchen was not large and therefore required minimum movement between drawers, oven, sink and pantry. I noticed that in bigger kitchens I got exhausted carrying and ferrying things back and forth, and became disoriented by all the swivelling and turning required to negotiate a larger space.

Looking at beautiful objects, pictures, paintings, plantings or patterns was helpful, too. I learned to let my eyes rest on some satisfying subject and stay with it far longer than I would have in the past. And then there was listening – to the sea as it flowed back and forth on a beach, to cicadas filling the air with their busy sounds, to bellbirds and morning skylarks, to the reassuring light hum of voices in friendly conversation. Touch was also important – feeling beautiful materials, Lui's warm woolly fluff, the smoothness of rocks heated in the sun on the beach. And I remembered the experiences of the past, visiting them in my mind and visualising places and people I had known, rerunning the movie.

Twenty-six

Then it was February 2005, a year since my bang on the head. So where had this journey taken me? What were my current capabilities? What did I expect?

I could walk for longer and further before I was overtaken by weakness. If left alone I would be fine in a familiar environment, such as at home, on the beach or in a small known shop, or in my office or Mark's office – depending on noise levels and busyness. I could last longer before I needed a rest. I could read a book; it took longer and I tended to repeat stuff, but I could complete it. I could talk for longer and with more animation.

And I was living each day, filling it with meaningful activities, having dreams again and working towards their fulfilment. I was loving my family, my children and their partners, celebrating their achievements, delighting in my grandchildren, rediscovering a new relationship with my husband and companion of thirty-five years. I was aware, open to the experience of life, waking each morning to a new opportunity to live a new day. I was so lucky.

20 FEBRUARY, 6 AM. *In seven days we will celebrate the marriage of young friends. I will wear the pearls again.*

I have just seen my husband off to the airport, en route to meetings in Tokyo. Last week it was Australia, next week his destination will be Amsterdam. The significance for me is that I have sustained the build-up days, the preparation with him, without collapsing, and this morning after an alarm not gone off and a prearranged taxi wake-up call not happening, despite these emergencies, I remained calm, helped him finish packing and stop panicking.

I walked down through the garden to the bottom entrance in order to farewell him. I walked back alone to the house, made a cup of tea, turned off the lights and climbed back into bed.

We are both turning our separate ways. After one year of me being dependent, attached, needy, I am looking forward to a year of regaining my old ways, independence, travel, home activities, reintroduction of work, reintroduction of social life, reintroduction of the more physical aspect of roles of grandmother, mothering, of companion to my mate, and most of all an emerging new confidence again of being able to cope again alone.

I look outside and see the light creeping through the trees slightly later each morning, hear the sea birds, noisily calling to each other, feel the stillness in the air and see the flatness of the sea. It is that time of year again, autumn here down under.

Just heard from the bellbird. They're slow this morning. I'm looking forward to the new day. I'm one of the lucky ones.

There will be no miracle. There will still be limitations, but I'm on my way.

Twenty-seven

It was November 2005 and I was in Townsville again. Ten months had passed since I had written those words 'I'm on my way'. Yes, I was. There was a way to go yet, but the achievements throughout that year had been enormous.

There were losses, too, and they were ongoing. The loss of independence was still very real. I'd adjusted to taxis. They got me from A to B, but of course I couldn't be spontaneous en route. It wasn't like the old days – my social life was really non-existent.

Visits from people were less frequent. When I did have people around, although I loved it, I was exhausted afterwards by the excitement. I still didn't enjoy loud, noisy environments, which cut out a lot of restaurants, and live music was fairly impossible. Movies were okay as long as I wore earplugs to dampen the soundtrack, and concerts – well, it depended on the composer and where I was sitting. But it was much more tolerable than it had been eighteen months before.

I was still using the walking stick, mostly for unknown and complex environments. Places like shopping malls and airports still threw me completely. I could walk unassisted in quiet, straightforward places and around any house I was in, but I was using a wheelchair at airports to cope with the distances through check-in and customs, and to the gates. Although very humbling, this giving in to being assisted made all the difference between being disoriented and exhausted, and arriving at my destination feeling relaxed and able to cope physically.

My tolerance for family life had risen a lot, though it still wasn't what it had been before. I lost patience rapidly and said so if two things were being demanded of my attention at the same time. I was still short on tolerance when let down by others or doubted. My confidence and security in my old roles had diminished greatly, and I battled for understanding of who I now was in the eyes of the world.

It was good to be a grandmother, and wonderful to have more time to focus on the little ones, but I still lacked my old stamina. My needs – for quiet, for rest, or just to be alone – had become vitally important.

I thought often of my own grandmother and of the relationship I had had with her for so many years. She gave me the gifts of love, of interest and focused attention, of delight in the sharing of ideas, of pride in my achievements and, particularly, of my intellectual activity. She gave me the role model of strength of opinion and fearlessness in the face of opposition or chaos. She gave me courage to believe in my abilities and in myself, and to forge my own path. It was this attitude that had helped me through some very lonely and rough times over the past two years. I hoped I could provide some of these qualities for my grandchildren, as well as maintaining my own interests and activities so that I, too, could remain an active, contributing grandmother.

14 NOVEMBER. *Still having vestibular troubles each day. Affected in the car by this. Cannot walk in a straight line while looking from side to side. Still cannot cope with two things at once. Still need daytime sleep or rest at least.*

17 NOVEMBER. *I'm so improved, but then still have problems. I'm different, my capabilities are different. Sometimes I can let myself panic, realising my limitations and wonder where I'm headed, but mostly just delighted by all of the pleasurable moments.*

Twenty-eight

It was the waiting to get better – like Estragon and Vladimir as they waited for Godot, distracted by Pozzo and Lucky for a short while. I could relate to the flies knocking themselves against the skylight in their frustration to get out to the evening light, trapped by the warmth of the house. I read somewhere that conscious waiting was enervating and therefore weakening. Trying to remain unconscious of the waiting was the best way to go.

Well into 2005 my eye still jammed shut and went dry when I was tired. I felt a pressure in my head at times, and pain where the holes were when I experienced a temperature change, such as getting into and out of hot or cold water. I also suffered when I encountered conflict or when I pushed myself in any way – too much talking, walking, writing. If I burned off energy on domestic activities, I had none left for anything else.

One night I had a dream in which I saw people trying to help me escape a stalker who was threatening my life. In order to assist me, they had to do things that discomforted me hugely and put me at further risk. According to them, however, there was no other way, so I had to trust them. There was a group of special police agents and a dog – an enthusiastic, trained but young dog that, in the event of my being lost or kidnapped, was supposed to be able to follow and find me. The problem was that it was out of control and kept lunging at me. I knew I had to stay calm and not panic. At one stage in the dream it had my wrist gripped between its teeth but did not puncture the skin. There was a woman in the house who was removing all stimulation and connection with the outside world. The television, the video, the telephone and the locks on the doors were being tampered with and made accessible only to the team. I arrived in the place of the dream in a plane with just me and the pilot, who negotiated the landscape at an extremely low altitude. It was breathtakingly excruciating and frightening, but I knew I must trust in him totally.

On waking, I felt that this dream related to all I had been through: my injury, my operation, and my submission to fate and the hands of others.

Twenty-nine

It was January 2006. In two weeks' time it would be two years since the whole thing had begun. I was a grandmother once more and would be again this year. The garden had altered and grown. It had improved enormously from the changes and additions I made during the first year after my injury. The house had also benefited from my caring and watchful eye. My business had slipped away, so quietly that hardly anyone had even noticed. All those things that used to give me such a rush of adrenalin, such a feeling of achievement, had subsided. I had finally cut off the landline to my office in town. When an eager young enquirer on the phone had asked about joining the casting agency, I replied, for the first time, 'I'm sorry, I had an accident and I'm no longer running the agency. I can't help you.' It had felt like a relief but also sad – another closure.

I had just found out from the ophthalmologist, after doing some base tests, that no, I would not be driving again in the near future owing to the ongoing effects of parietal lobe damage and vestibular difficulties. So the dream of independence extended again. I'd been going through a lot of testing with the head-injury assessment team, which had shown up my continuing difficulties while also confirming that the strategies I'd developed were, in many cases, helpful and innovative.

Those who had said it would take two years for major recovery to take place were right. What an impossible length of time that had seemed, like being given a jail sentence. How could I possibly survive two weeks, two months, let alone two years? But here I was, still moving forward, enjoying some of the aspects of my former life and discovering new paths that fitted better with my day-to-day limitations.

My physical strength was increasing, and because I was continually pushing the physical limits, my fitness and body tone were returning. Diet in these last few months had been important, and losing kilos I'd collected with all the lying around had been great for my self-esteem. Clothes bought during the rehab ordeal had been taken in and clothes bought before the accident could be worn again.

Life was different. Some days I craved to be in charge of my life again in the way I once was, driving my car alone through the countryside, feeling the wind on my hair and face, seeing the countryside flash by. I still dreamed of running, moving my body effortlessly through space. Mainly, however, I was planning new activities to fill my days. I struggled to hold together bonds between family and friends, and I was tentatively reaching out to new friendships. Sometimes I was just grumpy all day. Sometimes sadness swept over me. But mostly I was busy and content.

Thirty

Travelling had always remained something I was sure I would do again – and not just to be near family and friends. Yes, I'd been to Australia during the first two years of my recovery, initially with the full support of a caregiver or friend and then with my husband, and then on my own with airline support and family and friends at either end. But I was hankering after my old independence.

It's hard to explain that loss. You don't feel it at home in the familiar environment. After year one, I felt quite comfortable within my own environment and I was more independent at home, but getting out into the wider community was a different story. No longer in charge of my day, I had to find a way to make myself feel I had control and choice. This process has happened very gradually and I'm not aware of thinking out the strategies; they've just developed.

First, I found a taxi company I felt very comfortable with. The style of driving, the quality of the cabs and the discretion and understanding of the drivers – all these were important. For a year after I started using taxis I had many different drivers. I then started to use two or three drivers more regularly. The advantage of this strategy was energy conservation. I wasn't continually having to explain myself or fill in the half-hour drive with polite talk with a stranger. I could have a great conversation with the driver if I felt so inclined, or equally he or she would respect my tiredness.

Because I felt more familiar with, and trusting of, the drivers, I would take bigger risks when I got to town, pushing myself to try walking greater distances or going into shops on my own. I was never frightened; I just couldn't do things.

Then, towards the end of year two, I decided to set myself the task of going to a conference in Montreal. Long-haul travel, and then a schedule of commitment at the other end – how would that be? After nearly two years, aeroplane travel itself – sitting on the flight – was no problem, providing of course all the strategies were in place: earplugs for noise, sitting as far forward as possible to lessen the effects of any turbulence, and seated by a window so that I could 'hide'. I'd also learnt to pluck up the courage to ask noisy neighbours to turn down the volume on their headset. And, as I've mentioned, a wheelchair was essential at the airport.

Accompanied by a colleague as minder, I flew first to San Francisco, where I was picked up by a brother-in-law. There were difficulties with traffic, and the motorway trip into the city was frightening and confusing. Sunglasses helped, as did looking straight ahead.

A small, quiet hotel had been selected – perfect. It was difficult, however, explaining to exuberant pre-teenage nieces that Aunt Rosie couldn't participate in too much excitement immediately and needed some peaceful time-out.

Walking to the nearby restaurant wasn't really an option. A car was required even for two blocks. But determination spurred me to achieve my goals in San Francisco: buying dress-ups at the Walt Disney store in Union Square to fulfil grandchildren's dreams, and spending part of the day with family. A supportive brother-in-law's arm and assistance with the bewildering assortment of net and glitter did the trick with the shopping, and then we followed this with a family lunch at an Italian restaurant. Over-stimulation was the major problem at this point, so I needed the hot bath treatment, the lavender oil and quiet meditation.

After a sleepless night, it was early to the airport to catch a flight to Montreal with Air Canada. This time I was alone, as my colleague was on another flight via Chicago. I remember a feeling of huge achievement that I was on my way back to my old life. After a very difficult start in Montreal I managed to find a routine that worked. One of the hardest things was seeing all the people from my past. As usual, I was bewildered by people looking different and was much slower with initial recognition. I was also quite lost at first with the pace of conversations and the intensity of discussions. It bewildered me and I would retreat to the hotel room.

At first I ate my meals in my room as I couldn't work out a safe option, but this changed a week into the stay when I located a café very close to the hotel where I could buy delicious simple food and where the staff were supportive. I used this café as a meeting point, and found that I could invite one or two people at a time for an early dinner and have a reasonable catch-up. The café was also quiet, which made conversation possible.

Sharing a room with a colleague was fraught with difficulties, and many times I regretted that I'd made this choice for economic reasons. My fragile state became more obvious when I had to accommodate the needs of a relative stranger. My requirement for silence, for total lack of stimulation in the room and for regular food, and my inability to be spontaneous, all became a burden for my room-mate and her reactions felt threatening to me. So it wasn't easy, but we did it.

Again, the long hot soaks in the bath, the swimming in the hotel pool and the rest times all helped to keep me going. I managed to attend many theatre productions as part of the conference, often sitting alone at the back, ready to flee when I'd had enough. I found a taxi service that would drop me off and pick me up.

People were puzzled by my condition. I was shown compassion and kindness but essentially I felt very alone, as always. I was in a different location but the same problems remained, and a carefully planned timetable was essential to the management of each day. It was interesting to see what this did to my old relationships with international colleagues. I could sustain brief times with full-on conversation and then would have to withdraw. Those short periods of connection led people to believe that I was there with them – my old reliable, capable self – but then I would fade out and probably not follow up on conversations started. Ideas being discussed became irrelevant in the face of my drive to survive the rest of that hour or day. The projects dreamed up, the links made, could not be sustained. Was I a fraud? That was how I thought I must look and that was how I felt.

This has remained a pattern. I have the urge to be part of something – a dinner, perhaps, or planning a project. I begin with great vigour and excitement, my brain is active and I'm involved. Then I become aware of discomfort in my head and body. My consciousness shifts from outside to inside and my interest in the external diminishes. I know I can't deliver.

But I still don't stop throwing myself at the wheel. My inclination remains to keep going for the big connections, for passionate verbal sharing with other human beings, for strong debate over issues and values, and for the sharing of laughter and joy – the rewards from such connections don't leave my consciousness. So, despite all the setbacks and the sensible options to make my days more comfortable, I still head for stimulation.

Invariably, however, I end up offending someone. They perceive me as my old self. I go along in that vein for a while, then come to an abrupt halt and have a desperate urge to leave. If circumstances don't allow me to leave promptly, I become 'difficult' and am perceived as ill-mannered, uninterested, abrupt, rude, intolerant, spoilt, selfish. I probably am behaving in this way, but I don't intend to hurt or offend others. I'm just trying to survive.

Even with family and with close friends, and even after all this time, these perceptions are still pervasive. There are remarks such as 'Pull yourself together', 'Stop playing games' or 'Get a grip'. However, with work colleagues or students there is no personal emotional bond, so a distance soon develops.

On my side this produces instant paranoia: they don't like me any more; I'm no good as a colleague, a teacher, a director, a financial strategist; I'm no longer respected. That's how I feel at the time. I'm sure I'm still capable of performing well and have something to contribute, but it isn't sustainable or reliable. I'm liable to let people down.

Thirty-one

We read so much about brain injuries, about the accidents that cause them, about the aftermath and about the rehab, but not a lot about the specifics of what you can do for someone who has been affected in this way, what they can do for themselves, and what therapists can provide by way of support and advice.

The families and friends of those with head injuries constantly want to know when their friend, mother, father, wife, husband, daughter, son, will be fully restored. When will he or she be as before? When? When? When?

These questions, of course, have no immediate answers. They're left hanging there with a variety of responses from a variety of health professionals. 'In another year,' says one. 'Well,' says another, more cautiously, 'you'll feel better than you do now, with careful management of your life.' 'But,' says another, 'you may never get to be how you were before. You will, however, continue to improve.' These are evasive replies, yet at the same time they are honest attempts to prepare you and your family and friends for the next part of the journey.

The group of health professionals who are there to help you on your road to recovery are therapists, including speech–language therapists, physiotherapists, neuropsychologists and psychiatrists. It's quite a process finding what suits you and your circumstances, and it's never quite like your other life, where you would choose a health professional to go to. If your injury was the result of an accident, your therapists come to you through the ACC system. At first you're too ill to care much about who sees you, and the faces simply come and go. Then you begin to be more like your old self, and you want people who you feel comfortable with to accompany you on this journey of rehabilitation. My therapists talk to me and to each other, and to ACC. I'm fortunate indeed.

The therapists are there to assist you, encourage you, reassure you and challenge you, but in the end you must participate fully in your own rehab at the level and pace that best suits you. In hospital, the physiotherapist assisted me first with walking, helping me learn to cope with stairs and steps, and with early attempts to deal with everyday living independence, such as bathroom and kitchen activities. At that stage, just three or four days after my second operation, my big achievement was to walk supporting myself along the wall of the corridor and to make a circuit of the neurology ward.

In my first weeks at home I don't think any therapists visited at first, and I just attempted to bumble my way back to my old life. One day during a crying episode (these became more frequent), I found in my wallet the card from the hospital physio, who also worked privately. It was a Saturday, I think, but I rang and she said she would come to see me. This call began the whole process of involving therapists in my life.

I cried a lot after that initial session, so humiliated was I that a stranger was coming to my home in that capacity. I'd tried to make muffins to serve with the morning tea – after all, that was a past habit to welcome a visitor to my home. But it had been too hard, and then I was rapidly overwhelmed by fatigue from all the talking.

I was upset by my new situation in all respects. Yes, I wanted help to get back on track in my life, but no, I didn't want to be treated as if I was really ill just because my brain was exhausted and I couldn't move around. This didn't mean I wanted to be subjected to what I perceived as humiliating and childish tests. I resented being asked to rearrange my day, to make a timetable structured by the hour all day. I couldn't believe a stranger was coming into my house and telling me I should work out what we were going to have for our evening meal in the morning and make this a focus of that time of day. I felt like I was my mother, eighty years old. This was not me, a person who was so busy all day that a meal was the last thing I would plan in the morning. In my way of thinking, a meal arose from feeling hungry, from being inspired much later in the day – unless, of course, I was planning a dinner party, which would be fully arranged well in advance.

Since that first visit, therapists coming into my home has turned from a negative to a positive event. They get to see me in my environment, with all those influences, and they get to see how these might impact on me. The therapists who came to visit me early on in my recuperation all had the same general theme: that I shouldn't push myself, and that I needed to accept that for my brain to recover I had to stop quite often and for decent periods of time. It was also through my therapists that I got approval, encouragement and reassurance. I was led to a new way of looking at my situation. It was okay to feel overwhelmed and fatigued, and taking on little bits at a time was fine. They also reminded me that there were others out there on similar journeys.

It has been good to demarcate the week with appointments from therapists. Too many appointments and appointments that are too long can be overwhelming, but building good relationships with your therapists is important, so that you can trust them sufficiently to talk about your fears and frustrations, and your achievements too.

Those early therapy sessions were based around watching me move, improving my left leg gait and getting me to try to look from left to right. For many months I worked on looking just to the right, then to the left, and later I practised looking up and down while moving forward. At first these attempts would render me so dizzy and exhausted that I would have to lie down to recover.

After two years I was able to look left and right slowly while walking forward. I still have problems with looking up and down, and have to use a walking stick for balance when I do so. I walked on fairly rough surfaces from an early stage – around my hillside garden and on the rocky beach, for example. I believe this to have been useful for confidence.

The problems continued to be fatigue and balance issues. Therapist number one, a physio, was joined by therapist number two, a neuropsychologist, who was to work on psychological issues. I would talk and share my report of my week, saying how it was going with family and friends and what my goals were. These talk sessions were exhausting and sometimes I was very upset afterwards. But the visits from the two therapists, Megan and Clare, gave structure to my weeks, and their reports and plans gave me goals and showed me my achievements.

After some months the two therapists became three. I couldn't understand at first why I needed a speech–language therapist when I could talk, but she worked in many areas. For example, one of the problems that was acute for me during the first two years was an inability to focus on more than one thing at a time. If I was speaking to someone and a noise intercepted, such as a radio or another person, then I couldn't maintain the original conversation. The speech–language therapist did not do what her title suggests, but instead looked at appropriateness in planning the day and addressed fatigue issues. Also, if I was reading and put the book down and then picked it up later, it would be very difficult for me to recall the earlier information I had read. The problems were specific and subtle, and even identifying them with the speech–language therapist was useful. The neuropsychologist, meanwhile, aimed to assist with my emotional stability and with goal-setting and self-confidence.

By that stage in my recovery my week was demarcated with alternating visits from therapists and home helps. The days were very busy and sometimes I couldn't discern any progress. I felt like I was going in circles, dissipating too much energy on talking and planning, and on analysing time, rather than just getting on with the doing and being. In retrospect, I do think that you need to manage your therapy and recognise when it and your therapists are dominating your days to the extent that you don't have enough quiet time, or enough time to challenge yourself and find a path that suits you and your personality.

I was fortunate, in the second year, to have therapists who fitted well with me, my personality, my environment and my goals. In this sea of uncertainty and despair, I'm so grateful to these people for giving me hope and reassurance, and for reminding me constantly that I was going forward and that this wasn't an unusually long rehabilitation, that I was doing okay. I really began to welcome these therapy sessions as times when I could look back, look forward and show off my achievements. My therapists that year, Katie and Pat, listened and guided as we worked and laughed and cried together. Their ability to empathise and to be positive and calm was so important to me.

Keeping a close connection between the therapists, the ACC case manager and the GP is essential to the smooth working of the rehabilitation programme. At the request of ACC, at the end of each year I had to — and still have to — undergo an extensive assessment process with specialists, each of whom produces a follow-up report. The aim of this is to ascertain my therapy needs so that I receive the help I require. The assessments are emotionally draining and formidable, each lasting hours and stretching over several weeks or even months. They look closely at what happened — in other words, the accident and surgery — what followed in the way of ongoing symptoms, and what I am now capable of and what I am not capable of.

The resulting reports have both fascinated and horrified me. I want to pretend it is not me – I am determined that I am going forward to being the old me again. I think I found the reports particularly distressing to read because they outlined the identifiable problems. The more I woke up to my situation and the more I started to participate in the world outside my house again, the more I realised my limitations. It didn't pay to dwell on this. My days always worked best when I focused on doing what I was still good at, not on what I couldn't do.

In the third year following the accident and the surgery, my therapy slowed right down. Following reports from the neurologist, the ophthalmologist and the ear, nose and throat specialist, it was decided that physio wasn't helping and that the old brain stem damage, which was causing my giddy vertigo-type symptoms and visual disturbances, would respond best to quiet and rest. The symptoms abated for several hours following a shut-down period. However, they never fully left and would return in a very powerfully debilitating way when I was placed in a stressful emotional situation or a highly stimulating environment, such as when trying to cross a road, or cope with a busy airport or a loud, sparsely furnished café with a wooden floor.

As a result of the reports, my ongoing therapy during the third year consisted solely of neuropsychological support. There continued to be a lot to adapt to. Just having those session appointments written in the diary was important, like a stocktake, a reassurance. And the improvements continued.

I think I was very fortunate early on to have my high pre-injury functioning acknowledged. In her paper 'Key ingredients for successful rehabilitation from traumatic brain injury', published in the *New Zealand Journal of Occupational Therapy* in 2004, Anne Campkin wrote, 'High functioning clients tend to be measured as "normal" though their losses are greater and don't we know it'. An occupational therapist, Campkin had sustained a head injury and wrote this paper during her rehabilitation. Her conclusions resonated with me: 'As rehabilitation providers you can make an enormous difference in our lives. I believe that providers are merely facilitators. As facilitators you can give inspiration, ideas, knowledge and support to help us achieve success. Any success belongs to the clients.' She spoke of her own four years of struggle and how this success could never be measured in clinical terms.

For me, the providers who had the most positive impact were those who carried out the role Anne Campkin described. They were the people who came to our home and supported and inspired me to persist with my journey of rehabilitation, to come to terms with any new circumstances I faced. They were the people who didn't question the validity of my injured state. They showed respect for me and my changed circumstances, and my previous life. It was a life they hadn't known, except through summary forms, but they accepted it as having been a full and high-achieving existence.

As the statistics show, many marriages and relationships founder following a brain injury. A major part of the therapy I continue to go through involves maintaining relationships with friends, family and my partner.

I look back at my bewilderment, my grief, my fear at my new situation and my anger at my partner. I so much wanted him to know my loss and to feel my discomfort, to understand my frustration. My therapists would continually tell me, 'It's not him who's changed, it's you. You can't expect him to make those adjustments rapidly or even ever. This is the man you married. He's who he is and you're no longer who you were – make strategies, adapt.'

For at least two years I was so angry with these sorts of discussions. The bastards, I thought, how dare they. He has to change – I can't. Gradually, however, I've made some concession to this idea. It was my psychiatrist – vivacious, energised, committed – who managed to get Mark and me to look at what we were doing to each other. She managed the remarkable task of making us feel heard, both individually and together. She managed to make us feel celebrated as a couple and as individuals. I felt her understanding of, her empathy with, my situation. She took us from the muddle of now and the looking back, to looking ahead and going there.

My relationships with my children had become ignited and fragile at times. My psychiatrist validated the awfulness of the situation and then we moved on through it. She helped us to overcome what people said, or what we knew they were thinking but not saying: 'You look fine', 'You don't look sick', 'That's just part of getting older', 'Oh, that happens to me all the time'.

My psychiatrist helped to diffuse the anger and the grief. We discovered the humour. She encouraged us to celebrate what we still had. She allowed us to accept that we had been through a particularly challenging time, separately and together. We came to realise that I wouldn't get my old life back, because I'm not that person any more. My current therapists encourage and support me in using this transition in a positive way. There are days when we can even enjoy the 'new' me.

As part of my journey in writing this book, I asked my family and friends for their thoughts.

AIMEE (DAUGHTER)
The biggest thing I noticed is that my mother went from being fiercely independent and very, very busy with enormously high energy levels compared with other people, to being more fatigued, more vulnerable and childlike in her emotional state — more needy — losing the independent part of her personality. She still desired to be independent but didn't have the capacity. I observed grief and a sense of loss.

If I'm at a needy place in my life when I want to be nurtured, it's very sad for me because my mum is no longer strong enough to be that person. My role is to be mother to her, i.e. she needs to lean on me physically. I find that weird, extremely stressful. As a child you want the parent to be there for you. Then the rug gets pulled out from under your feet – we have to be there 100 per cent for the parent.

Then there was the fear that we might lose her. How was she going to come out of it?

The trauma of being in a hospital environment, around the other tragic cases, for me, it put things in perspective about how fragile our existence is.

My mother and I have always had a tempestuous relationship. When the accident happened I stopped thinking about my own issues and focused more outside myself, on her situation. Coping with brain injury is not so tangible, and it is difficult for an adult child to deal with. At first at least she did have holes in her head and her hair shaved so I could go 'ooh' and it looked awful. Down the track, when she looked normal, it was very difficult. If a brain-injured person is displaying inappropriate behaviour or acting like a five-year-old or being extremely needy you can forget they've had a bang to the head. It's hard not to get angry and think, 'Why are you behaving like that?'

My observation, with both my mother and my husband, who has a head injury, is that some aspects of their personality have been exaggerated, and this can be challenging for the family. You've got to rise above it – put your own needs aside. From my mother and my husband's perspective – they think other people have changed.

MARK (HUSBAND)

At the beginning when Rosie was wheeled away I felt so alone, so isolated. I held a lot back that I wanted to share with her and couldn't. Her availability changed and she became more demanding in ways that she never had been before.

It's very difficult when your wife becomes a different person and she doesn't think she's different.

There are changes in terms of mobility and energy levels. Many times I thought my companion was a very elderly person.

There's a greater sensitivity and vulnerability in her.

There's no longer the same balance in terms of negotiations because of your partner's neediness. Whereas in the past there would be negotiation about apportionment of work, now your partner has the final trump card: 'I'm not well and this is what I need.'

I felt pity for my wife; this was a different relationship, something new. She was imprisoned by her condition and the way out was a long, difficult passage. The passage kept extending further and further as we proceeded along it.

I was scared, too, when Rosie experienced pain in her head, worried that it might happen again.

My partner is still essentially the same person, yet in many respects also distinctly different. Rosie was incredibly socially active, with about five lives running in parallel – this shrank to one life focused primarily on her own needs and rehabilitation. Other interests came then, but there was no longer a focus on the wider world. She had always been engaging, but now seemed self-absorbed and preoccupied. We used to do lots of stuff that was fun and now we just repeat simple routines.

Three years on we have adapted and developed new areas of shared celebration and experience centred more around the home.

MISCHA (SON)
I'll start with some positive things. A side effect, as a result of being home with time on her hands, is that her cooking, which was always good, has improved tenfold. She's got more time for all of us. Even though she's distracted by her predicament, she's available more for talking about any old stuff, which is a change – we never had that before.

The negative things are that she's more frail physically and mentally than before. It's frustrating. Her brain is still busy with ideas but she doesn't have the capacity to carry them out. She often gets pretty frustrated.

I was expecting a full recovery after the first operation. After the second, I started to get really concerned. From then on, I realised she was turning over a new leaf in her life – for better or worse. It was a situation none of us had any insight into, but we do now.

There should be open discussion in the early stages. There was a lot of *fear at first. People shy away from discussing things to do with the head – the mind in general.*

OLLIE (SON)

I felt pretty guilty in a way because when I came home and saw my Mother that day, 12 March 2004, I knew she was seriously ill and no one, including me, had done anything about it. I was angry with her as well for not telling anyone or pushing anyone about how sick she had been feeling over the last few weeks.

Mark was away so I took Mum to the private hospital where a brain scan had been organised. It was so surreal. I had a pit in my stomach. I thought Mum was going to die. She was obviously scared and so was I. But when the doctors came and said she had a bleed in her head I knew it would be okay. I'd seen this sort of thing on television a lot and people have these haematomas and seem to be running marathons the next day, if you believe the tabloids! So it was scary and I knew she could die, but the reassurance was that at least it was operable and at least she didn't have a tumour, which had been my worst fear.

After the scan at the private hospital, the nurses said to get to the hospital fairly fast. I'm still surprised they didn't order an ambulance for the hospital transfer, considering the situation. We got in the car and drove to the hospital.

The first operation went smoothly and the doctors reassured us that everything was going to be ok. Although the doctor did warn us that there was a small chance that the bleeding would reoccur.

During the first operation, it all happened so fast that I was on autopilot and running on adrenaline, plus I don't think I realised the severity of the situation. I was all right for a couple of days and then I had a bit of a breakdown – emotional overload.

Sure enough the bleeding did reoccur. Before the second operation I was really worried. I didn't want the bleeding to continue and for her to have more operations. They were invasive surgeries. I was pretty upset and bloody worried. It was very difficult seeing your mother like that, not once but twice.

I was distraught about it but I didn't really have many people to talk to about it. Nobody really understood what was going on. If you tell people that someone's got a bleed on the brain, but it's okay, they can operate, then everybody relaxes and thinks it's going to be fine – different from 'My mum's got a tumour and nothing can be done about it.' People seem to grade these things in different classes, which is fair enough, but at the same time this situation didn't really get the empathy from other people. They just seemed to think it was going to be okay. People underestimate brain injuries.

Anyway after the second operation I was a bit of a wreck. Aimee, my sister, came and that was great because I couldn't bear to go through it again by myself. I hated being at the hospital and in the neurology ward. It felt quite a sad place – to me, anyway – and pretty upsetting.

After the second operation I kind of accepted what had happened and how Mum was. I didn't really think she would recover quickly. It wasn't like she had the flu or some other minor ailment. She had had brain surgery, which by definition is fairly major. Just because she was discharged from hospital did not mean that she was 'better'. She was very ill in hospital and she was still very ill when she got home.

Despite the fact that Mum and I have had a tense and fraught relationship at times, and that there are things about her both before and after the operation that piss me off, one thing is that I really admire her strength. I can't believe how positive she has remained and how much energy she has – although she can be over the top and a bit of a drama queen. I really admire her tenacity and continued optimism that she has maintained throughout her sickness.

I know that a lot of people would be in a different frame of mind faced with Rosie's situation, and mentally how would they cope?

After the surgery right through until Michelle began to help, I had tension between guilt of not wanting to help because I wanted to do my own stuff and knowing I needed to help. It has been very difficult being relied on so much. The dependence thing is hard.

MOTHER

I was shocked – she seemed to be indifferent. She looked older and very sick. I grieved because I didn't know what to do. She didn't seem to want to communicate. She seemed to be in her own world. This thing that had happened to her took away the joy of sharing.

She seemed like a stranger, very internal. She looked old and so slow.

I kept thinking, What can I do? It was hard to know how to comfort her. She didn't want to talk about it. I couldn't understand what was happening to her.

SARAH (FRIEND)

When I came back from the Chathams I arrived at the hospital from the airport as Rosie was being prepared for surgery. She said to me, 'I've got to go and have this stupid operation. I'm going to be all right tomorrow.' She was anxious about the operation and about the outcome, but she was going into it with the feeling that she was going to be fine. The expectation was that she would be up and about relatively quickly.

In the early stages I thought of Rosie's condition as convalescence and I didn't really have any idea until well after the second operation that it was actually going to be a lot different. She was really sensitive to noise, so we couldn't have music on. She was really sensitive to light, so it couldn't be too bright or too dark. She really appreciated food, though: she hadn't lost her taste buds. She got very tired and was sensitive to temperature change. She could no longer concentrate on complicated conversation. I suppose I thought all this would get better within six months or a year, and Rosie would be back to where she was.

She became frustrated about not going out and not seeing people, and yet when she did go out it was harder and noisier and rougher, and she wanted to hibernate. She was always pushing herself well beyond her limits and frustrating herself in the process. It took Rosie two years to be able to manage her tiredness, her energy, but not to stop striving.

The other thing I've found really difficult is that after about a year, people would ask me, 'How's Rosie?', expecting her to be better. Some people would understand the process of recovery from a brain injury: most were sceptical and thought she could have been malingering. I had to explain to people that in actual fact she wasn't and that it was going to be a longer process because brain injuries are tricky things. I found on the whole that people didn't really understand. Most people would see Rosie when she looked great, because as soon as she felt she was going to crash she would go home or go to bed. I know her very well and would see her change, sometimes very quickly. I felt I had to make constant excuses for Rosie and her behaviour. People would ask, 'Is she ill?' or 'Is she being difficult?' I had to explain that it isn't a matter of just getting better, that recovering from a brain injury is a slow and often frustrating process that takes a toll on the patient.

Often visitors would see Rosie at her house and think she looked great, because she would prepare herself for their visits, but as soon as they went she would crash. I started to recognise the stages as she would get quieter and quieter and begin to go grey. Even now, after nearly three years, her face changes quickly from looking very sparkly and animated to exhausted, with dark rings under her eyes.

I noticed other changes in Rosie's behaviour. She became less tolerant. Her mannerisms became accentuated, e.g. she was more fussy about food and less tolerant about it being wrong. The same applied to people and situations. She would say, 'Right, I can't deal with that' and leave abruptly, whereas before she would have been more sensitive or more challenging and deal with an issue. After three years she understands her limitations better now and knows how much rest she needs and when to stop. I guess she pushes herself to different limits now – she has changed the boundaries. She is more subtle about her intolerances and knowing when to stop.

Recovery has been a gradual process. I've seen her go through grief and frustration, when the recovery process seemed to be taking longer and longer. Extreme grief like that which Rosie has gone through resurfaces from time to time – the loss of a certain style of living and of experiencing life. Friends feel powerless to help because maybe one has to deal with it oneself. In that situation, or in any loss, one needs to let go of expectations of how one thought one's life was going to be lived and have to rethink every project. Will it get any better? We don't know.

ALISON (FRIEND)

Rosie and Mark came to Australia to visit us about six months after her brain injury and operations. We had talked on the telephone frequently before their visit, when she was able to hold the handset. Often calls would be cut short because she could no longer bear the buzzing in her head from the exertion.

This is a person we knew as a dynamo. She had always used the telephone as her instrument to speak to the world, to contact her friends, to connect with her theatrical associates. Now here she was looking slight (still beautifully dressed) but wearing a woolly Rasta hat to hide the half-shaven hair and to keep her poor head warm. But what shocked us most of all was her panda eyes. Huge blackness encircled those lovely hazel eyes, which appealed for compassion and relief from the agony she was undergoing. Her movements were wobbly and uncertain, and she felt faint and dizzy frequently.

We admired her courage even to have embarked on the flight across the Tasman and up to Noosa, let alone the huge effort she was making to stay vertical and to stand on her own two feet, unaided. Being a great traveller (and often a solo one), Rosie found the thought of not being able to get up and go a severe blow; I felt the same too, as she was such a wonderful companion on 'girlie' trips.

And Mark, well, I think he was bereft without the Rosie of yore...his sparkling Rosie, who managed the household, children, animals, garden, three or four different jobs — including the running of her drama school — and their active social life. That Rosie was always ready with an invitation to dinner, cooking delicious food, and she provided a table that was rich with conversation and bonhomie. This time they both seemed to be struggling to communicate with each other about where they were going to go and how they were going to deal with the effects of the accident.

Determined to enjoy the bushland around our home, Rosie and Mark set off one morning for a walk. Mark strode the length of our garden, leaving Rosie wailing behind, hopelessly unable to keep up, crying in frustration and fury. I suggested she use a walking stick and persuaded her to borrow one we had here. She told me she had one in Christchurch but had left it behind because it embarrassed her. She had no intention of anyone ever thinking that she was old and infirm, believing that this is the general perception society has of anyone who uses a stick. I said to her that it was also a means to broadcast that she was unsteady on her feet to everyone who saw her with it, and that they would consequently make allowances for her frailty. It's obvious she's not old!

Conscious of providing calm, we also did our best to entertain and divert Rosie and Mark, albeit temporarily, from the enormity of this immense, life-changing experience. Living so far away and knowing that we could only play a tiny part of the ongoing rehabilitation process, it has been a delight to speak on the telephone and receive text messages. Later, in 2006, Rosie began to send little emails which, knowing the cost in energy it takes her to produce them, are a privilege to read. Alan and I have the greatest admiration for Rosie's strength and courage, and we deeply appreciate seeing how this event has caused both her and Mark to adapt their lives in a way that has drawn them closer together, increasing their love and respect for each other.

GARY (GARDENER)

I thought Rosie would get better quicker, but now I know. I've never come across this sort of thing before. Visually she looks spot on. Some people think she might be having us on but I know. She used to be out there tidying the garden with me, once a week, but then she would be out there for only twenty minutes to half an hour before she had to stop and rest. Three years on, she works in the garden with me longer, but she can't sustain more than one and a half hours without me saying, 'Have a rest.'

Maxine went into hospital in March 2004 for planned surgery to an acoustic neuroma. She suffered some complications in the days following the operation, which necessitated her being in a room on her own. I remember that, and she remembers me shuffling around to visit her there once. Then one day she had gone home and I was still there. It was not until months later that we saw each other again, but we spoke on the phone and found we could relate easily to one another, sharing how we felt. We had post-operative problems that were very different in some respects and very similar in others.

Maxine had terrible pressure headaches. But she could walk unaided, she could garden and after six months she could drive. She was completely deaf in one ear and had balance issues to deal with in relation to this. Like me, she suffered from the loss of her old independent life as a high-level support person in a busy academic institution. Like me, she had to adapt to finding her way again without the framework of her profession or the routines that old life necessitated. Like me, she was incredibly fatigued.

Occasionally Maxine would drive to my place – only a fifteen- or twenty-minute journey – and we would excitedly compliment each other on how good we both looked and tell each other how well we were doing. We would exchange stories of our new lives and the problems we now faced. We always ended our times together exclaiming how fortunate we were to be alive.

Our appearance is normal, but we suffer because people expect the old behaviour and response that we had before the surgery. They expect that you're not going to get emotionally or spiritually fatigued. But you need space, and quiet, and aloneness in order to recharge.

It's physically and emotionally very draining. People with head surgery are affected in every way. Where to from here? What does the future hold? Are we going to have to make a lot more changes? Is the transition now going to be very quietly unseen until we reach the stage of 'betterness'?

We don't have the same resilience that we had in our past life, of being able to work eight to ten hours a day and then come home and do things – that old life is finished. If we were in our thirties we might be thinking differently, but in our fifties we have to accept this situation.

Because you're not in paid employment, not socially recognised, you feel you're a failure. I feel I'm not worth anything because I'm not contributing. I saw myself as being a very reliable person – now I feel totally unreliable. And after being a really conscientious and reliable person it's very hard. People don't understand.

We're slowed down, but we have to adapt. Because essentially, we're lucky.

EVA (FRIEND AND HEALER)
I had never encountered anything like this before Rosie. Her hypersensitivity was very extreme. I couldn't even move my hand through her aura without her noticing it. I had to treat her very cautiously.

The person with TBI (traumatic brain injury) needs a peaceful, calm environment, with support but not too much stimulation.

In the early days post-injury the people who visited Rosie didn't seem to be aware of this need. She required love and support but she couldn't talk for too long or about things that weren't very relevant. It exhausted her. Family members and friends need to be made aware of this sensitivity.

Six months later people think, I've done my bit now. The TBI person is at home. They can cope. But that's not really the case because there are so many things such patients can't do by themselves – the ongoing support is essential. Rosie still quickly goes into overload. The most important thing is to communicate and tell people how she is feeling.

The medical staff in the neuro ward were very receptive to massage as a tool towards recovery. It is important that people who have had a head injury do get deep relaxation, so foot massage is very useful.

Alternative remedies are Rescue Remedy for trauma and arnica drops to help with the bruising. When you have an anaesthetic, the soul fades; afterwards, it needs to return and balance needs to be restored.

Rosie didn't use arnica drops for the first surgery but the second time she did, both before and just after the operation, and the bruising was significantly less. Rosie's hearing and smell were so acute. I had to be so careful never to come near the head for two years or more.

One of the most difficult aspects of my accident and subsequent operations has been the dramatic increase in my sensitivity to sound, light, taste, touch and smell, as happens to many sufferers of a brain injury.

We live our lives so often unaware of the five senses and their almost automatic operation. And our senses often become dulled because of stress and overloading. Most of us, as we grow older, take on more responsibilities, cramming our lives with them. We look to workshops and therapists, or to holidays in remote places, to try to retrieve those sensory experiences we remember back there somewhere in the mist of the past. But a brain injury can change all that.

I'd always had faith in my senses and 'listened' to them, so when I became ill it was a natural reaction to indulge them, and to rearrange how I indulged them to suit my new circumstances. In the first few weeks after the injury this strategy worked for me, and I believe this is a positive way for those who have suffered from a brain injury to help themselves and to be helped by family and friends.

When it came to my sight, I used sunglasses to cut out the light and concentrated on the beautiful. When I looked at flowers, I focused on the petals, the colour, the shape. This exercise can fill in a lot of time and is also a pleasurable experience. I found looking at the glossy photos in high-class travel and cookery magazines a comfort too. I'm a sensualist and a romantic, so perhaps these suggestions may be over the top for some, but they did help me.

I also learned to brace myself for the visual disturbance caused by complex designs and textures, such as the highly patterned carpets that are common in hotels and airports. Public bathrooms with many mirrors and doors were also disturbing and frightening places. But I kept on making myself face these challenges, with the support of my family, friends and helpers.

I have always liked indulging in the smell of delicious soaps and lotions – especially the wonderful, heavenly scent of lavender. Always a soother for me, using such items is now an essential ritual during the day.

The sensation of being touched through massage is another great healer. It must be gentle and soothing, from people you trust. Areas as far away from the head as possible should be worked on at first – for me, the feet and legs have always been safe. I've continued to have treatments from Eva, my massage therapist friend. These are times when I can be still and totally let go.

One of my most acute senses proved to be hearing, and I found that I needed to cut back on all sound in the early days of my recovery. It came as quite a shock to realise that I didn't want to listen to classical music, and that any music – always a comfort to me – was now very disturbing. In hospital, brain-injured patients should beware noisy night staff, unoiled doors and TVs blaring out loudly in other parts of the ward. At home, and later in public, it is helpful to minimise negative sound experiences as much as possible – wearing earplugs has been a huge plus for me.

The taste and smell of good food has remained an important part of my ritual each day. At first I began to concentrate on delicate foods that were both visually pleasing and flavoursome – brought into the hospital from local restaurants or a friend's home. I also ate cashew nuts, for strength, in those first few days after surgery.

Later, food shopping became part of my rehabilitation. At first it was the small shop owners who allowed me to maintain some participation in the food purchasing process each week. I'm so grateful to them. Relationships were maintained over the telephone. I placed orders; others picked up the food – this enabled me to continue my culinary interests and expand my cooking repertoire.

I extended the food shopping method to buying clothes and gifts. These exploits, first by telephone and later in person, have given me much pleasure. I commented recently to my neurologist that I felt guilty about the pleasure I got from visiting a beautiful boutique store and purchasing something. There was satisfaction, in the item bought, but mostly in the process of purchasing. This type of shopping environment – less busy, less noisy, less complex – and the pleasant interaction with staff, allows me to lose myself in the moment, and I feel a sense of achievement.

The neurologist suggested that these forays into the world, 'cotton woolled' as they were, should not be a source of guilt, but should be celebrated as achievements and as connections to my old life – unless, of course, I was being totally excessive or buying completely unnecessary goods. Now that last qualifier gave me lots of problems. What was necessary to me and my new world couldn't often be justified as necessary by my husband, who struggled to understand my new 'hobby'. I often felt ashamed, thinking how an action that used to be squeezed into my busy working week in order to feed or dress the family or myself, has now become a major focus of my life and a source of great pleasure. The purchases may be for me or for others – both are equally pleasurable. I have encountered much kindness from the retailers I have dealings with. They have given me marker points on this long rehabilitation journey. They have shown compassion and genuine pleasure in seeing my return to the world, and I've been moved and encouraged by them.

It was during year three that the telephone food shopping began to extend to actual participation. Saturday became the food collection day, with me on board. Poor Mark, how he must have dreaded those Saturdays – with me moaning about the car speed and getting frustrated at the local farmers' market when the live music accompaniment overwhelmed my ability to purchase food.

On those early visits I was overcome by the excitement of seeing and relating to so many people from my past in a friendly, informal setting. I would get exhausted and wobbly and not actually buy any food.

We persevered, and the market on a Saturday has now become a highlight of the week. Mark has become a full participant and the whole process, although taking a few hours each week, brings together socialising, restocking the food supply and being together – still struggling to understand each other's needs, but being together.

I gain in confidence when I have some minutes away on my own in the market area, though I like to know where Mark, my support person, is. We leave, the car filled with the smell of fresh basil and coriander and dill and some salted bread, along with various fruit and vegetable aromas. I've had my fill of social activity, and am dreaming of the recipes I'll make with the produce on board. Mark is probably thinking, When will this food collection be over so I can get back to the boat or work in the home office? But he has adapted and given me that feeling of independence.

It is during these shopping forays, whether with Mark or on the jaunts with friends or assisted by taxi drivers, that I gain more understanding of my condition, of my disabilities and, more importantly, of my abilities as they emerge.

Walking is another aspect of my new life that I have found difficult. I walked to the end of the hall with a friend just three days after the first operation, yet even now there are days when it is very difficult and I stop short, unable to go on – the message just doesn't get though. I've learnt not to panic, as the message will get through in time. It's like an electric socket that needs resetting following a power overload – it doesn't mean the power is off permanently or even for a long period. My power might be off for just a few seconds, but of course I can't push a reset button, and if I do attempt to move off after a couple of seconds my overload switch will just trip again. Instead, I have to wait until it resets itself – I'm not in control of the process.

Early on in my rehabilitation I also came to realise how important it was to have things to look forward to, and to keep on making plans but to be prepared to postpone or cancel them if I didn't feel up to it. In addition, I think it's important to maintain your appearance. Just because you aren't out and about doesn't mean you can't look good.

But the main thing to hang onto through it all is that with rest and routine and care, and just doing bits of the things you did before – taking small bites – things do get better.

Postscript

It's December 2007, almost the end of the fourth year following my surgery. Here I am in Bali, accompanying my husband, who is a delegate at the United Nations Congress on climate change. I realise how far I have come in this recovery process, enabling me to make such a trip. Looking back at my writing over the past two years, I reflect on the journey.

APRIL 2006

Some days I feel like a fairy-tale character who goes to sleep for a lengthy period then wakes and carries on as if nothing has happened. I'm in the city I've lived in for thirty years or more and yet I feel confused when I find huge changes to an area I knew well. How can this be? Is life an *Alice in Wonderland* trick? At times I'm puzzled and confused – I feel out of touch. And then in the car recently, after being in town too long, while waiting for the driver to collect an item en route, I looked up to see the road in front of me distort. It appeared as a hill, not as the flat road I knew it to be. Wow, and I didn't even pay for the experience.

There's disbelief if I think beyond the day I'm in – that I'm not my own boss, that I can't say to my body, 'We're going to go gardening now, you and I, and we will garden for two hours and then have morning tea.' No, it won't do that. Sometimes I can last for twenty minutes, sometimes half an hour, sometimes ten minutes. But I'm not in charge. My bed in the late afternoon is still the most inviting proposition. And quiet is still essential at this time.

I've just come to the end of an assessment process that has gone on for approximately eleven weeks. I've seen a team of brain injury assessors who are reporting to ACC, a neuropsychologist, a physiotherapist, a speech–language and an occupational therapist, and a vocational assessor. Then there was the ophthalmologist, the ear, nose and throat specialist, the neurologist and the vocational therapist. It was very strange looking back over my career, reviewing the past and then contemplating the future.

The assessments have been completed but the reports aren't all in yet. They all follow the same line. You have some damage from your three injuries: the fall, the first surgery and the second surgery. You may continue to improve but you will need to keep up the strategies you've developed in order to get through your days with the least possible distress.

My assessment of my current situation is that I'm much better than I was six months ago, but I move forward into this third year with awareness of my handicaps. I have limited energy levels, a limited ability to take in highly stimulating situations, limited tolerance of stressful situations, a constant disbelief, if I allow myself to dwell on the situation, that this is really me. I'm frustrated at my lack of mobility and freedom, at my separation from the work world. I hate the separation from family and friends sometimes caused by my need to depend on others to get me around. I can still get pale and faint, with ringing ears, sometimes even hysteria at times. More and more often I dream of striding along without any walking stick. It makes me feel euphoric when I wake up thinking it is real.

I got asked yesterday, as I often am, 'How are you?' 'What does it feel like?' Usually my assurances are brief and not specific, but yesterday I was feeling extremely fragile as I sat waiting for a taxi in town, after having negotiated a small task that I hadn't tried for maybe six months. A young woman who has lovingly asked after me on a regular basis these last two years of rehabilitation, said to me once, 'It's good for people to know how it feels – please share it.'

So here it is – not the big achievements of rehabilitation but the restrictions that are still there two years down the track.

In company, I can't participate in intense conversation for more than thirty minutes and I can't cope with multiple conversations. I have to wear custom-made musician's earplugs to block out noise and I try to converse focusing on only one other person. I can't bear music being played during conversation over dinner or, if it is being played, it needs to be what my children rudely call 'lift music'. I can't walk in town for more than a few metres without feeling drunk and wobbly and detached from my surroundings, and I can't cross busy roads easily. I can't look up or to the side without feeling an 'earthquake' effect. I can't travel in a car over ninety kilometres per hour on flat open road and fifty kilometres per hour elsewhere without feeling very uncomfortable in my head. I can't be touched around the neck or face area or head except by the hairdresser I know, and even then I can't bear any pressure on my head.

I can't attend a concert or performance of any sort without encountering a variety of problems, which display themselves according to the closeness, loudness, the type of lights and number of bodies in the auditorium, and where I'm sitting in a row. I've learnt to sit in the back of a theatre or in the first row if I'm upstairs. I wear earplugs and even sunglasses inside the theatre. Sometimes choosing whether to watch and not listen or whether to listen and not watch helps. It's all about trying to monitor the input. Sometimes I have to leave the theatre during a difficult or intense bit, or if it's too noisy or too light, and then I return. Sometimes I have to leave altogether, as was the case only two weeks ago at a cabaret event, where there was too much stimulation all around and in a small space. This shattered me for a whole day after the attempt and depleted my confidence.

On patterned surfaces I need a walking stick. In very highly coloured patterned areas I have to use a person's arm for support or, in the case of airports, a wheelchair. In the dark I have to look at the ground and be escorted, or look up to some light ahead and aim towards it.

I can't cope with more than two or three hours with people, even my grandchildren, without requiring complete silence and a lie down. And I still need two to three hours' rest in the afternoon. I can't run and I'm not permitted to drive. I can't keep to time lines on projects I've undertaken or telephone calls that need following up. I'm unable to use the computer for more than half an hour without feeling disoriented and sick. I can read only in short bursts and can't manage complex material. I can't control a rising temper or cope with intense passion of any sort for more than a short time.

The biggest progress came early in 2006 when Michelle arrived from Brazil. She wasn't a therapist, a chef, a housekeeper, a nanny or a gardener. What she brought to my life at this stage of recovery was quiet companionship and assistance in the many aspects of my life. She allowed me to be a full-time granny during periods of the year by assisting with little ones so I could enjoy having them to stay: she was a natural nanny. Michelle became a superb assistant in the kitchen, joining in the pleasure of creating good-quality, inventive food, in the garden and in the home office. She helped so ably and quietly and quickly in the kitchen that I was able to turn out great meals without exhaustion and even, with careful planning, do some entertaining again.

While Michelle slowly learned English, I began to take back some areas of my life – time and energy for stimulating conversation, some business phone calls early in the day, some liaison with Mark's office via Maria, our new office administrator. Maria's arrival increasingly allowed me to let go of work responsibilities

I had been holding onto. Things were going well, but every day I faced the limitations and the need to accept them.

And there was still the hurt caused by the attitude of others. I found myself in grief at times about why those closest to me could be so cruel, as I perceived. When I asked my daughter about it one day recently she gave an extremely useful and illuminating answer. Aimee, of course, has the added perspective of being the wife and partner of someone suffering a severe head injury. On July the 14th 2005, her husband HJ was badly hurt as a result of a car accident in Australia.

It seemed impossible to believe when we got the phone call while sitting in a café in Hanmer, where we had gone for a quiet two days. My poor darling daughter, seven months pregnant with their third child, having to cope with another close person in her life with a head injury. He was in a critical condition in the first hours after the accident. He sustained a fracture to the skull, which extended ear to ear but didn't require surgery as the bleed came out and wasn't contained inside. I was fascinated and horrified that someone else in my family should be embarking on this journey or anything remotely resembling it.

Seven days after the accident, my daughter-in-law Sol and I, along with my granddaughter Lili, set off for Townsville. HJ was stable and out of intensive care, so I figured I could help by sitting with the children while Aimee was at the hospital, and that I could assist with advocacy for her and her husband. Sol could be another support person and, most importantly, a driver, and we would cook! Arriving at the neurology ward in Townsville wasn't easy. I was deeply upset by seeing HJ lying there, so unlike his usual self.

It wasn't long before I realised how very different brain injuries can be. After the first week, HJ got up and walked quite vigorously down the hall. The physio came and got him. I went with them, aided still by my walking stick. The physio asked him to stand with his eyes closed. I was very anxious about him falling, which is what I did, and still do, when shutting my eyes. He, however, shut his eyes and didn't fall. I was amazed and then horrified at my own condition. 'Why doesn't he fall over? Why do I?' I found myself tearfully asking this physio in Townsville.

HJ had problems though – they were just different from mine. He looked stunned by his new circumstances, reduced to a state of dependency. 'I feel sunk,' he said. I felt his pain acutely and it brought back nightmarish memories of the loss of control, the enormous fatigue. As we sat looking at him asleep, his face hollow and absent, I asked Aimee, 'Did I ever look this bad?' 'Yes,' she said, 'you did.'

NOVEMBER 2006

But we move forward, changed by our new circumstances. Though back at work and achieving at a high level intellectually, and physically active and fit, HJ still has no sense of smell or taste, and he continues to suffer from enormous fatigue and inability to cope with more than work and family life without stress.

So Aimee had added insight when she explained to me that a stranger has nothing to lose by adjusting in the brief moments, in the short term, to a head-injured person. But for people who have an ongoing relationship to sustain, it is very threatening to their existence having continually to adjust to their brain-injured parent, friend or partner. When Aimee told me this I suddenly saw things from another perspective, and some of my anger, hurt and disappointment in the reactions of others abated. It must sometimes be so difficult to be around me. I remain stunned, however, by what I perceive as senseless, selfish behaviour when a slight adjustment can make all the difference to my coping with a situation.

For example, at a recent large family reunion, when the music was turned up suddenly, I clutched at my head and felt as if I was going to be sick and needed to leave. But I hesitated to leave – I had travelled a long way to get there and I wanted to be part of the celebrations. The person who had turned the music up was an older relative with a hearing impairment. It was hard to get him to understand my needs, that I wasn't just being difficult or a demanding drama queen. When I told my elderly mother about this incident later, she said, 'Well, he did have a point. Why should your wishes be met when there was a whole room full of people who also had needs?'

I screamed at her, 'But I've had a brain injury, a brain operation. Doesn't this count for anything, for any consideration, not even from my own family, when I've made such an effort to get us all here? Don't I matter at all?

'I was so devastated I wanted to disappear – never to see any of them again. Don't they know what I've been through? Don't they know that small adjustments to their behaviour can make all the difference to me being able to be there?'

It was like a dream I'd once had. Two young people who knew me well, whom I'd trained and launched into careers in the media, were saying, 'Look at you, there's nothing wrong with you. You look all right, you look great. What's all the fuss about? No, I haven't been to see you, I haven't offered my support. I'm quite angry actually because I don't see anything wrong.'

I lost it emotionally. I threw myself onto the young man who had been coldly analysing me, scratching, clawing, kicking and screaming. Then I broke down into sobs, saying, 'I've had a brain operation. I might look okay but this did happen to me and I'm still having problems.'

I can vent my anger like this, in real life or subconsciously, but others don't change, and why should they? It's me who has the problem. I just have to use strategies. I so look forward to invitations, but every time something is too hard I cause problems and discomfort to others by requiring them to adapt to me. Often I want to give up. Increasingly, others seem to feel that I'm somehow using my injury in order to be more demanding and difficult.

Again my daughter explained it from her perspective. As individuals, we want things to be comfortable for ourselves: this is just human nature. The difficulty with a head-injured person is that you can't see anything wrong. After the initial trauma of seeing your loved one or your friend injured or recovering from surgery, you slip back into a belief that everything is okay. And then you're reminded by the person's behaviour or demands that it's not all right. At that stage you feel like retaliating. It's not nice to be confronted by vulnerability. It's difficult to be given that responsibility. As Aimee said, 'You never were vulnerable to us, the kids. You were strong and independent. We weren't used to you being needy. So it seems now almost manipulative, like a performance in fact!' Suddenly some of the comments people had been firing at me made sense. I saw why the grandchildren seemed more 'there' with a little shoulder, or a hand, than the big children.

There continues, however, to be a small number of adults who willingly offer a shoulder, an arm, an outing; who coddle me, who allow me to join in with life and can offer subtle support while still enjoying the essence of the old me. These are the people who don't judge, who celebrate, though it is changed, our ongoing friendship. They offer loving care and companionship when I want it, quiet and solitude when I need it. They don't push but allow me to go at my own pace, telling me to slow down when I'm overtired, recognising my condition, yet not dwelling on it. They provide remnants of my old lifestyle, while not commenting too much on the change and celebrating my achievements. They let me know I'm attractive, that I'm achieving, that I'm interesting to be with. They offer intellectual companionship at an intense level but withdraw discreetly to another level, or altogether, when I begin to fade – without making me feel guilty or a failure. They're just there when I'm distressed, not out of duty but out of love. They let me know, when appropriate, that they have a sense of my loss. They have fun with me, while accommodating my subtle changes in ability. These are the companions I'm comfortable with, safe with, and inspired by. I thank them all.

Some people went from my life – it was too hard – and some people came into it. Rebecca was one of those newcomers. She carried on what Sarah had started – those trips over the hill, not to a medical appointment, not to a work trial, but just for a 'jaunt', as these trips began to be labelled. Always a great pleasure and huge boost for my confidence, these trips, first with Sarah and then with Rebecca, became a very important part of my rehabilitation. This pleasure has continued and the jaunts are always different – nothing too demanding, not rigidly set each week, gradually enabling me to expand the boundaries of my contracted world.

During my rehabilitation, I had found ways to bring comfort and rest for my brain and had developed strategies to block out disturbing stimuli. For me, these gradually evolving routines were part of my recovery strategy, but once again my daughter had another perspective. When she was staying recently, I asked her, 'Why don't you talk to me about your own life?' 'I can't,' she said, 'because in the evenings [presumably when we would have talked], you watch TV.' It's true: I use the television to take time out at night, something I never used to do. I had never considered that this new behaviour would affect my children.

As Aimee explained to me, when a brain-injured person indulges in some new behaviour, whether it is watching TV, turning music down or off when they used to fill their life with music, or telling grandchildren to be quiet when they used to cope with the hubbub, it is a harsh reminder that their loved one has changed. This is discomforting. It's a reminder that the effects of this injury are ongoing and not just tidily diminishing.

The way I see being alive now, from the place I am in, is more or less as follows. First, it is fabulous to have the opportunity to be alive and stay alive. Second, the practicalities of it, and mastering the practicalities, still appear to be hugely challenging on a day-by-day basis, and the only way through seems to be to adapt to the moment.

APRIL 2007

Lately I've been feeling like it was time to leave behind the brain issues – that phase was over, I thought. Now I can move on to non-related projects. I don't want to carry those issues, those disabilities, with me for the rest of my life. But then every day I keep going in a circle with any new project I attempt and keep coming back to what seems like unfinished business. Once again, I have to come to terms with the fact that I do have an ongoing disability, and that it does affect my whole life and how I enact it.

Every day I continue to be affected by others in ways that disturb as a result of my heightened sensitivities. Every day I disturb others by these heightened sensitivities. Every day my fatigue levels and inability to control my emotional states, whether they be positive or negative in nature, remind me, pull me back. Hey – slow down – hold on – you can't keep up this pace – you can't get that excited – you can't handle that conflict – and so it goes on.

These are the ups and downs and complications of life in a world with people and happenings outside your control. Living with my family and them living with me has always been a challenge. I would say this has been the case right from the beginning. Looking at my young granddaughters now, I see that strength and determination, curiosity and stubbornness that drove their parents to the edge and over it at times, and I remember what I might have been like at three and four and five.

Living with others is always a challenge, even when all the circumstances are optimal, but throw a traumatic brain injury person into the mix and you come up with some very 'special' challenges.

My poor daughter, in absolute frustration following yet another brief attempt to have the traumatic brain injury mother to stay, exploded with the statement, 'Great for you to have written a book Mum, I'm pleased for you, but it's really me who needs to write the book about what it's like to live around a brain injured mother.' There was an enormous explosion of anger and tears on both sides – each party feeling severely hurt, and it took a few hours and days to recover, and then on we go, to try again, never giving up because we are family and we do care about each other and we want to maintain the contact.

And it doesn't go away. You're driving now, you're so much more independent, you're making major decisions, you can have the grandchildren to stay, you go to the movies, you go out to dinner, you talk on the telephone and send emails. But hang on, there is still something very strange. This new you, going about these tasks and these activities – essentially it is you, but a different you. It's strange, too, for those who love you and live beside you.

To get the day started – that is the key – without getting too overloaded and too over-stimulated, without offending or being offended, without feeling unsafe and making others you are responsible for feel unsafe, without losing your cool because the person you love doesn't fit into the routine you have devised. That horrible choice you have to make – do I carry on being in this situation of relating to people, continuing the activity, whatever it may be, or do I retreat into a quiet spot on my own with little structure, where I can feel safe, uncluttered, but often so lonely?

God – when will it ever end? Sometimes a panic sets in and there seems no way out, no way forward, no way to escape, and I get so tired of explaining. It's a strange new world. Hardest hit are our partners – those people who remember us how we were – in my case a very spontaneous person, unafraid of sudden changes to plans, always able to adapt quickly and now, here I am, going raving bonkers if my plans and routines aren't completely adhered to. It's especially difficult when I've been on my own for a few days or weeks, and then my partner returns to what had been his home too, and now it's a monitored space.

My main objective every day after nearly three years is to take comfort from the discomfort. To have the least time feeling weird and out of balance and out of control. I am still triggered easily into terror by incidents that remind me of how bad I felt. For example, yesterday I had been carefully rowed from near to the shore on the beach, further out to the head of the bay, with two granddaughters on board. We stopped and landed so they could enjoy the rope swings hanging from the willows. They invited me to sit on the bar attached to the rope, which I did. I tentatively swung and then did two more. It felt odd, but freeing, and then the weird head stuff started. Very soon I felt extraordinarily awful and went very pale, according to my husband. Worse was the feeling of powerlessness and inescapability from the disruption to my balance system. In that moment I went backwards again to the beginning.

Every day I must plan, and realise I am changed in my tolerances and therefore in my capabilities.

Most of us don't like dealing with conflict, but coping with conflict and dealing with it after a traumatic brain injury brings a totally new set of circumstances. Conflict, or even the suggestion of it, is terrifying for me now. The minute a voice is raised or lowered in anger, the minute the face looks slightly changed by anger, the second the voice on the other end of the phone sounds cold, I am filled with fear, my breathing changes, my legs become heavy and my being feels like it is shutting down. If I allow this response to continue, I will become quite immobilised. If I feel safe enough, such as when I am with my husband, I can fight back. If I am with anyone else, I disintegrate gradually, usually to tears, even if it is with someone professional in a formal setting such as a legal office, accountancy office, bank, or talking on the telephone to customer services representatives. If the conflict is with my partner, my rage lets loose. I am ashamed of the escalation of my indignant anger and the havoc it can cause. For someone who does not like loud sounds anymore, I sure can make them when I have been set off in a rage. The after-effects of these outbursts are quite catastrophic on intimate relationships. People who love me and are closest to me are horrified by my loss of control. I am rendered ill – head dizzy and hurting – by this display of anger, and a distance comes between me and the people I need most to nurture and love me. All round, the situation is a disaster.

Time alone seems to help me retrieve these shattered relationships – periods with no stimuli, no telephone, no music, no input. Just sitting, nursing my wounds. A few expletives shared with only myself also helps to diffuse the situation. I then try to think how it must be for the other person, and try to distract myself by doing something very simple. Just looking at something – the first leaves of the grapes, sparkling with droplets of water from last night's rainfall; steam rising from the cold, wet roof as the morning sun strikes it; and Lui curled in a ball at the foot of the bed.

NOVEMBER 2007

It's been a busy early morning. Its only 7.30 AM and I'm already exhausted and ready to go back to bed. It's this endless cycle of not having any energy left over after life delivers its daily dose of happenings that makes me so frustrated and at times very sad. It is an isolating experience, and alienating. Instead of kissing my husband goodbye this morning I withdrew – stormed off – with an 'I can't cope' attitude. My day to me is an unbearable mountain I just can't face tackling again. But here I am an hour later – back in bed, eating my breakfast. My husband has gone to his day's activities, which include talks with an MP, a flight to Wellington for meetings, return to Christchurch with a business colleague from Brazil, dinner here at home and preparation for a flight out tomorrow to the US. I will try to still myself, and know that if I take plenty of breaks today, lying down with no stimulation, I may get the tasks I have set for myself done.

How do you go on waiting and waiting for the heavy legs to go away, for the balance to return, for the tolerance to sounds to increase, for the day to come when you can stay up all day? I wonder how people in prison cope, staring at walls all day, every day – what keeps them going? In all those stories of incarcerations down through the ages, was it hope that sustained them: thinking that someone would release them, that an earthquake would bring the walls down, or that their jailers would have a change of heart? Or were they overcome by a slow, creeping madness so that they no longer felt the need to live in different circumstances?

We inhabit a noisy planet. Even in the quietest places, there is always sound. A fly buzzing past, birds excitedly communicating, wind in the trees, a distant hammering of a building being built: these are pleasant sounds, but on some days even this is just torture. Tuesday was so full of sound my legs did not want to carry me. The neighbour had at last begun the tree-trimming job we have been begging for over the past three years. An assortment of chainsaws and tree-munching devices filled the area with loud, harsh noises, but this was sound in the middle ranges. It seems to be sound in the very low registers and at the high frequencies that cause the terrifying disturbances for me. A leaf sucker, for example – a cheap version; that is torture. I am driven to seek sanctuary from the sound in the furthest rooms of the house, and still I cannot escape totally. Then there is the sonic-type booming sound from 'boy racer' cars as they speed past at all hours of the day and night. My thoughts range from 'I want to hide, to run, to get away', to 'I want to stop the sound.' A walking-stick attack does come to mind quite frequently.

And then there is the problem of waiting rooms. It still amazes me how medical establishments catering for unwell people can fill their waiting areas with sounds of a crass nature, such as talkback radio stations or infomercial TV. I also find telephone calls difficult when I am put on hold and subjected to commercial radio, radio talkback or very loud music. I find I cannot keep the receiver close to my ear. I feel the anger and upset rising, and one of two things occurs: I either hang up, ring again and tell the person about the inappropriateness of what they are subjecting the person on hold to; or I leave the receiver lying there, forget, and miss the person finally taking the call. Either way, it is distressing.

Then there are people noises – conversations that get too loud, in restaurants, at the next table, amongst family, and particularly loud children noises. Before this brain injury happened to me, I do not recall consciousness of sound like this. Keeping myself focused on only one sound also becomes difficult if there are two competing sounds – for example, minding two grandchildren simultaneously is extremely difficult. Loss of energy and loss of temper in these situations is almost inevitable.

In July Michelle left. It feels very strange getting my independence back again. I know it's still a limited independence compared to the old life, but it is something I longed for during the period of time I spent being heavily dependent on others. So here I have it – independence – but what can I do with it? I have a car to drive, a day ahead, lists to make, things to achieve. It seems easy, it seems exciting, but it's not quite like that. Take driving, for example. Following testing in April I was given approval to take to the road again. If I am well rested and have had plenty of fluids before I set out, I feel safe driving at first. The fatigue sets in after about twenty or thirty minutes. The symptoms range from my breathing becoming more shallow through to sharp head pains and a lot of yawning. I must stop, put the seat back and have a bit of a lie down, or go somewhere and have a cup of tea and a rest. The scope for full independence with the car is certainly limited by these problems.

Independence means I can create my own plans for the day and for the week. I can make social commitments, work commitments, family commitments. At first it was so exciting to know I could go to town unaccompanied. I could go to lunch with a friend. I could stop off at a café and read a paper – only I could and I couldn't. I feel like a child finding my steps again, not entirely confident to go out there all alone. Not yet, I tell myself, but soon. I still dream repeatedly about going out without the walking stick, and I still look at photos of myself in the album pre-accident, pre-surgery, without the walking stick. Perhaps it is just a habit I tell myself, perhaps I can do without it. But this stick of mine is now part of me, my reassurance that I will have support in the world out there.

Meditation helps to slow me down. I watch the leaves rustling on the huge poplar outside my window, or a small bird, a silvereye, hopping delicately among the grape stems on the pergola below. I discovered an amazing method for calming the brain quite by accident. I had picked four tulips from my garden. They were a rich buttery cream colour but closed when I picked them. I put them in the cream jug on the old oak desk at the foot of my bed and watched them. They were so beautiful in their bud state, full of promise. The first morning after I put them there, they were open slightly, but the weather was cold and grey and they stayed like that all day. But the next morning, the sun came out and warmed them. I watched as they slowly opened. It took about an hour for the first opening to occur. I went away and when I came back they were fully opened, showing dark brown centres, yellow stamens and cream interiors. Gorgeous. Late that afternoon as I lay having my rest – the prerequisite to savouring the evening – I watched the process in reverse, when they closed up again for the night. I enjoyed this show for eight days before it was over and the tulips had finished. They had to be thrown away. That will do me for a meditation.

The ongoing problem for me, the head-injured person, is twofold. First, there are my very real difficulties, which take over when my brain has had enough; second, there's the judgement and lack of understanding from others and the need to explain myself continually. Sometimes, in the light of others' reactions, I even doubt my own handicap. I see my family, all preoccupied, marching off ahead of me across a tarmac runway towards a small plane we're about to board, and I think, 'Hang on, perhaps I haven't got a problem here. It's just determination and I'll get to that plane unaided.' And then a noise from an aircraft, a pattern on the tarmac, and I'm slowed down or stuck. No, I'm not being overly demanding or trying to get attention, I simply need assistance if I'm to get on the plane. To me it seems so simple – as simple as needing a drink of water or going to the bathroom.

It's a balancing act, keeping a semblance of the old life while my rehabilitation continues, remaining connected while not overloading myself; keeping intellectually active while not freaking out; retaining and celebrating passion while not becoming over-stimulated; maintaining some social life while not getting exhausted and offending or cutting off friends; making my partner feel loved and cared for when I'm screaming inside for more understanding and empathy.

I need to find space and peace within a busy family and work life without losing my temper or being seen as too demanding. I need to sort out, too, when I should refer to what I'm still feeling as symptoms, and when I should ignore them and pretend for the sake of a social situation. Is it still appropriate to mention my situation? As I build up my exercise regime, when have I done enough, or too much? I have a good life, a rich life, but it's a different life. I think, though, I have stopped waiting and started just being.

So here it is, my offering to you, the reader, of a journey not planned or wanted, but a journey that many others with brain injuries will recognise and, I hope, learn from and find solace in.

Acknowledgements

Special thanks to:

Mr Martin Macfarlane and the neuro-surgical team at Christchurch Public Hospital, whose interventions saved my life.

Dr Philip Parkin, Dr Debbie Mason, Neurologists; Mr Philip Bird, Otolaryngologist; Dr Anne Young, Psychiatrist; Dr Clare Botha-Reid, GP; Dr Murray Smith, GP; Debbie Snell, Graeme Clarke, Megan Phillips, Neuropsychologists; Katie Hodge, Pat Hopkins, Clare Jamieson, Buffy Devlin, Tracy Partridge, Therapists; Rhonda Wicksteed, Triscia Tubman, Training support; David Moxon, Jeanette McBrearty, and Liz Brenen, along with other nursing staff of the Neuro-science department; Anudarma Marshall, Didier Le Guen, Osteopaths; and Eva Mason, Natural Healer.

All of you have listened and cared and helped me with your healing skills to move me through a very difficult time.

Graham Menary, CEO BIA (NZ) Inc, Rebekah Loukas, BIA (NSW), and Harley Pope, former CEO BIA (NZ), now retired, who read the manuscript and gave encouragement.

Dr Roger Rees, Emeritus Professor Disability Research, School of Medicine, Flinders University, Adelaide, for his powerful endorsement and belief in the manuscript.

Dr Lutz Beckert, Respiratory Physician for your support with my medical school teaching

Miranda Van Asch, Barbara Larson, and Richard Webster for their enthusiastic response and guidance with the manuscript.

Jeanette Stanley for her calm encouragement, her typing skills and for finding her way through my notebooks! Maria Cropper and Joy Hussey for their administrative skills and patience. Carol Fletcher, Antoinette Cossar, Hugh Matthews and Wayne Bailey for professional business support.

Leigh McPherson, Rick and Debbie Smith, Hank and Aprilla Jacometti, Simon and Nell Pascoe, and Tim Barnett and Ramon Maniapoto for your friendship and support.

Ishy Walters and Michelle Santana whose patience and commitment to helping me get my life back on track was amazing.

Lavinia Araya and Gary Kennard for helping to 'keep the home fires burning' and to all who have helped and continue to assist on the home front – most recently Kim Saltero and Anne Mackay. I am so fortunate to have your assistance.

Carl Watkins for his retrieval of, and continuing perseverance with, the hair style!

Suzanne Stagg whose help facilitated my return to air travel.

ACC staff Suzanne Rowe, Jeanette Meldrum and Heidi Gwynne for your sensitivity in dealing with my rehabilitation.

My wonderful editor Anna Rodgers for bringing order to my manuscript when my disorderly brain could not.

Robbie Burton and the team at CPP for your belief in this manuscript and making the book happen.

The friends who hung in there through the challenge of it all, there are many of you – thank you, especially to Sarah Lovell-Smith, Philip King, Rebecca Garside, Paula Middleton and Alan and Alison Pearson for bringing beauty and light to my constricted world.

Those in the wider community for your patience, encouragement and kindness, you helped me get 'out there' again – thank you.

My dearest family:
My children Aimee and partner, Mischa and partner Sol, and my son Ollie, who went through so much in the process of supporting me. You have given me a purpose.

My darling grandchildren Reuben, Sophia, Arlo, Lili, Grace and Iñaki for the joy you bring me.

My mother Eileen Roper and mother-in-law Margaret Belton for your wisdom and caring and to all the wider family circle who cared.

But most of all to my husband Mark who has gone through it all and is still here with me and for me. Thank you dear Mark.